Prais

MW00880031

"This is an extraordi   .n healing by an extraordinary man. He shows himself throughout as a powerful, intelligent, strong yet compassionate fighter with incredible focus and a herculean drive that allowed him to break through barriers and a determinate refusal to take no for an answer. He pushed himself well beyond where others might have yielded, with a singular focus of wanting more time with his wife and children. They fueled his drive."

~Dr. J. Michael Marcum, Psychiatrist

"When I first heard Doug's story, I thought what a great inspiration for those facing serious illness and their care-givers. But this is a story everyone should read, as it contains so many insights and lessons for living, and done so with humor, courage, faith and always hope. Thanks for sharing your story, Doug. It has now become part of mine in the most meaningful ways."

~Rev. Bass Mitchell

"Doug Gestwick's *Do Whatever Is Next* is a love story, and more. It's a story of confronting, receiving with grace, and moving through cancer. And it's more. It's a story of love for music and poetry, and more. It's a story of faith, and more. It is ultimately that most real part of our soul's journey when the heart cracks and breaks, until it ultimately breaks open to God and life. Doug has a gift for story-telling, and for sharing the wisdom of ancients in that most real of voices. If you've been searching for a memoir beyond cliches and bumper sticker slogans, read this, read it again, and take it to heart."

~Omid Safi, Professor in the Department of Asian and Middle Eastern Studies, Duke University

"As a pastor, I have accompanied scores of church members and many other friends in their fight to defeat cancer. Some have emerged victorious, achieving remission. Some have transitioned to life after death, with resurrected bodies. But all have been profoundly changed by the invasion of cancer cells not only into bodies, but also into family systems, and affected loved ones. Among all the beautiful and courageous cancer fighters I have known, none have been as fierce as Rev. Doug Gestwick. This man determined from the beginning of his diagnosis that he would conquer the cancer beast as it invaded his body. I am deeply moved and inspired as he shares his story. His fight, faith, family, and friends emerge as worthy companions for his journey. After five years, he is STILL STANDING and FIGHTING!"

~Charlene P. Kammer, Bishop,
The United Methodist Church, Retired

"Doug takes us with him sharing the critical decisions he makes as he navigates his mortality; from the perspective and understanding of a Pastor. He deals with the many needs of his congregation and family as a man facing a type of cancer with no known cause or cure; given a diagnosis of 14 months to live (Stage IVb Mantle Cell Lymphoma). He exudes faith in his approach, which is believing when you don't see, obeying when you don't understand and persisting when you want to give up.

My former career as a professional football player for 12 years, many of those years in Doug's hometown of Buffalo NY with the Buffalo Bills, provided an understanding of pain and how to deal with it. Doug talks about the conditions and experiences of enduring all types of pain. His courage and dedication to his family and congregation has not and will not let him quit. His Never, Never Quit attitude as he explains, is down to the cellular level of his being, he talks to himself on the cellular level.

His education, training, and commitment over his many years as a Pastor has enabled him to derive tremendous energy from his life's commitment to his family, friends, and congregation that he truly is a Blessed Man!

If I had to use one word to describe Doug's journey, it is that of a Hero striving to complete in this lifetime, his commitments to his family, friends, and community. His pursuit of commitment is a tribute to the sanctity of the human spirit."

~Lou Piccone #89
Former professional football player

DO WHATEVER IS NEXT

SurThriving After a Cancer Diagnosis

Cover and book design by Pat Murphy, Pat Squared Design

For more information, email authorddg@gmail.com

ISBN: 9798448371707

A portion of the profits from the sale of this book are being donated to Massey Cancer Center at Virginia Commonwealth University in Richmond, VA and to MD Anderson Medical Center in Houston, TX so that these two great institutions can continue to Do Whatever is Next.

*To the five people I need most in this life;
my wife Clara, and our four children,
Ryan, Taylor, Brandon, and Laura,
I dedicate this book.*

*I have fought as hard as I have fought,
simply and solely because I wanted
another day with you.
You gave me reason to want
to live another day,
and not to just survive,
but Thrive!*

*You all are my world,
and what a beautiful world it is.*

Contents

I Am From…

I am from churches
From stained glass windows and hymnals

I am from services
Perfect attendance and participation
Listening well and singing loud

I am from gatherings
Many faces, I've never seen them all
Knowing my name

I'm from questions
People asking me how I am and how
I'm doing

I'm from caring faces
People knowing all my situations
And asking my opinion
Thinking 'cause they know my family
I'll open up to them

I am from waiting
From "his numbers are good" or
"He's worried cause they're low"

I am from fighters

And I am from survivors.

~Laura Gestwick, 2017

1

Whatever is Next, Do That!

*The people you most need in life will appear
just when you most need them.*

It's been said that your entire life can change in a moment. That is true. Mine did.

What follows is "my story." We all have stories. We *are* our stories. You are your story and I am my story. My hope is that by sharing my story you may connect with it, and in some way make it part of your story.

June 8, 2016. That was the date of my second conception. I thought at that moment it was the beginning of my descent into hell. I was wrong. It was the beginning of a new, richer, fuller and more meaningful life.

It was the day I was diagnosed with Stage IVb Mantle Cell Lymphoma. (MCL). I was at a meeting of the newly formed Board of Directors for the Virginia United Methodist Assembly Center, which was a decrepit property that had "reverted" back to the Virginia Conference of the United Methodist Church when it went out of business and its entire board resigned. We were in the midst of electing new officers, and trying to figure out how to unload this money pit when my cell phone rang. Recognizing the number as being that of my gastroenterologist who had performed a colonoscopy on me several days earlier, I left the room and took his call in the hallway.

"Mr. Gestwick, I am very sorry to be doing this over the

phone, but this can't wait. The results came back from pathology and you have Mantle Cell lymphoma."

"What is that?" I asked, as the hallway started to spin and my world collapsed in on me. I distinctly remember telling myself to breathe slowly in through my nose and out through my mouth. "MCL is a very rare form of non-Hodgkin's Lymphoma, with no known cause, and unfortunately, no known cure," was his reply.

"OK," I said, not knowing what to say, "What do I do next?"

"Well, that's why I'm calling. I made an appointment for you tomorrow morning with an oncologist here in town. Good luck Mr. Gestwick, you're going to need it." And with that we ended our phone call.

I walked back into the meeting room where the conversation sounded to me like Charlie Brown's teacher "wah wah wah…" I then did something you should *never* do if you get news like I got. I googled "Mantle Cell Lymphoma". I had no idea of what was going on around me, my world was getting smaller and smaller as I read from the Lymphoma Research Foundation:

> "Mantle Cell lymphoma is typically an aggressive, rare form of non-Hodgkin lymphoma (NHL) that arises from cells originating in the "mantle zone." MCL accounts for roughly six percent of all NHL cases in the United States. Frequently, mantle cell lymphoma is diagnosed at a later stage of disease and in most cases involves the gastrointestinal tract and bone marrow."

My heart was racing, my mind was spinning and I felt like I was suffocating. I had to get out of that room, out of the building, and away from people—*fast!*

I got to my car without having to engage anyone in conversation, and I just sat for a few minutes. I had no idea where my life was going, where my family's life was going, but I knew that in that instant *everything* changed. That was June 8, 2016. At that moment I did not even know how to dream of being at the place in life I am now. The Doug of this moment is totally unrecognizable from the Doug of that moment. I wouldn't wish what I have gone through on anyone. And people look at me like I'm crazy when I add—but I wouldn't change any of it either.

I texted my wife Clara and asked her not to go to the "power band" class at church, and to be home when I got home and to not call or text me. Then I called my brother. He was in Philadelphia with his son for a Louis CK evening. I told him I would talk to him later. I then called Dr. Kim Schlesinger, an oncologist who had been a member of my church before she and her family moved to Northern Virginia. WH Auden once said "one of the greatest experiences in life is meeting the right helper at the right time." For me, that was Kim. She stayed calm and was extremely reassuring throughout the phone call (which I really needed—thanks Kim!). I told her who I was seeing the next day and she said, "No, if you were my family member, I would want you to go to John Kessler. Let me call him for you." She did, and Dr. John Kessler has been my lymphoma doctor ever since.

About an hour later I pulled in my driveway and ran upstairs to our bedroom, shut the door, and slumped into my rocking chair. I burst into tears, and after what seemed like an eternity, Clara came in. She took one look at me and asked what was wrong.

"I have mantle cell lymphoma" I told her.

"What is that?", she asked slowly, a lump visibly forming in her throat.

"I have no idea" I told her. "But it's rare and apparently deadly."

And with that, not knowing what to do next, we just sat and held each other and cried. That was probably the best medicine I could have had at that point. Pierre Teilhard de Chardin said,

"One cannot progress in being without paying a mysterious tribute of tears..." Payment was beginning.

That night, we fell asleep holding hands and crying. Or I should say, eventually Clara fell asleep. I didn't. I have always had trouble falling asleep. It seems when my body goes horizontal, my brain kicks into high gear. And was it ever racing that night. I didn't know what to think about, or where to begin. Like a Ferris Wheel, I was going round and round with no real idea where to get on or off.

I knew I had to tell the children, the church, and our families and friends. I was not looking forward to any of these. Our oldest child Ryan and youngest child Laura were both living at home, although Ryan was planning to move to Holland semi-permanently, as soon as he could get the proper authorizations. Laura was still in high school. Our second son Taylor was away at the University of Virginia. Our youngest son Brandon was on a year-long cross-country road trip with his childhood friend Emerson. I didn't want to tell any of them over the phone; I wanted them all to hear it in person so I could see their faces and be able to hug them. I also didn't want a few days to elapse between when I told one of them versus another. My preference was to tell them all at the same time, although I didn't think that was going to be possible. I also wanted to tell them before we said anything to the church, or to anybody else. For hours I played the possible conversations over in my mind, trying to find exactly the right words to convey the terminal diagnosis I had gotten.

I had to change the narrative going on in my head, so I made a vow. I vowed that if one in a million beat this thing, I was going to be that one person! I had spent my children's entire lives trying to teach them how to live well, and now I had my last teachable moment as their father. I was going to teach them how to die well.

I have always been a meticulous planner, and a long-term planner. For thirty years I had planned mine and my wife's retirement. Clara and the children would be well taken care of financially for the rest of their lives. In fact, the day before, Clara and I hit our number. Financial planners tell you that you should have a "number," a figure to strive for with retirement savings. We had hit that magical number the previous morning. That same afternoon a package arrived in the mail for me. It was from the world-famous cellist Yo-Yo Ma! As I approached my 58th birthday Clara and the kids asked me what I wanted. I told them I didn't want any *thing*, but if they really wanted to get me something, to get me cello lessons. I have always loved the cello, and in particular Yo-Yo MA. They did, and at the young age of 58 I started learning to play the cello. On a lark I decided to look up Yo-Yo MA and see if I could find an address for him. In minutes I had it and wrote him a letter telling him how much I admired him, and how much his music meant to me over the years. I really wasn't expecting anything back. But there it was. He had signed and sent me five of his CDs along with a note taking me up on my desire to someday shake his hand. Retirement number hit in the morning, five CDs from Yo-Yo Ma personally in the afternoon. Life couldn't get any better right? That was June 8. The next day came the call with my diagnosis.

As I lay in bed and thought about these two striking contradictions within 24 hours I made some decisions. When life seems out of control, you can regain some of that control by doing what is in your power to do. The phrase "do whatever is next" came to me and stuck. The universe gave me the very bit of advice I needed in that moment. Do whatever is next. That one mantra was going to get me through a lot of trials in the coming days and months, although I didn't know it at the time.

I was reminded of a quote from Rumi that also came to me that night.

"The moment you accept what troubles you've been given, the door will open."

I didn't know what that quote meant then, but I do now. In this book I will use the name/term "God" and "Universe" interchangeably as my reference to Divinity, knowing that many of my readers will be of a different "tribe" (As Leonard Sweet likes to say) than me. In your head you may leave it as I wrote it, or you may substitute God, or Allah or Gaia, or any other higher power. The Universe has many truths to share. But they are not revealed to the merely curious. Extensive work on true self is necessary for each precious truth to be revealed.

I've spent the better part of my ministerial career teaching people that authentic prayer is not about asking God to change our circumstances (how most people and most church's pray), but asking God to change US, in the midst of our circumstances. Most Western Christian prayer is medically based, (just listen to almost any church or see their prayer list), and asks God to change the circumstance of the one being prayed for. Can God reach down and perform a miracle? Of course God can. Will God? Probably not. But somehow, we've convinced ourselves and others that if we pray hard enough, or often enough, or loud enough, or quiet enough, or get enough people to pray, that God will reach across the firmament and change our circumstances. This is just a set up for heart ache and possibly turning against God. However, if you change your focus, and instead of asking or imploring God to change the circumstance of the one you pray for and instead ask God to change *them* in the midst of whatever is happening, you will hear and see an answer to your prayer that is much more real and authentic than when you plead to God to invoke a miracle.

I prayed that God would indeed change *me*, through all of what I was going through, and grant me the grace to be the best husband, father, pastor, friend and fellow traveler in whatever time I had left. In addition to vowing to be the one in a million who beats this thing, I vowed I would not in any way be a "victim." I was going to have a positive attitude, believing that our minds have powers we aren't even aware of. I can't heal a cut on my finger. But yes, I can. I don't know how to heal a cut, but my mind does. My mind and body have healing abilities that I am not able to articulate, or consciously manipulate or use. But I believe those powers are tapped into more readily when one has a positive outlook. I vowed I would look for the positive in everything, no matter what I had to face. And as I learned along the way on this journey, not all storms come to disrupt your life, some come to clear your path. You're allowed to be disappointed. You're allowed to be angry. You're allowed to be scared. You're allowed to cry. But you are not allowed to give up. NEVER give up! NEVER EVER give up!

The morning after my diagnosis, when my feet hit the floor, I turned to Clara and the first thing I said was, "You know what today is? Today is a GREAT day to be alive!" I decided that would become another sustaining mantra, and it has.

A beautiful day begins with a beautiful mindset. When you wake up, take a second to think about what a privilege it is to simply be alive and healthy. The moment you start acting like life is a blessing, I assure you it will start to feel like one. Time spent appreciating is time worth living. You are only responsible for the effort, not the outcome.

There is a *lot* to do when you've been given a cancer diagnosis. Whatever was next, I was going to do it.

Preachers have a phrase for Sunday morning. We call it, "the relentless return of the Sabbath." No matter what else is going on, (births, deaths, marriages, family issues, etc.), Sunday has this uncanny ability to show up, like clockwork, every seven days. And you better be ready.

Sunday, June 11, 2016 was an excruciatingly challenging day. We had not yet told our children, so we had not told anyone. We didn't want word to leak out to any of our four children, who would be devastated enough when they heard it from me. I sure didn't want them hearing it from somebody else. Clara (who worked together with me as the associate pastor) and I had to pretend all day that it was just a "normal" Sunday, when "normal" no longer had any meaning.

Thankfully, the week after that was Annual Conference for Virginia. The United Methodist Church is divided geographically into Conferences that get together once a year to hold our business meeting, adopt the conference budget, and on the last day of conference "fix" the appointments for the coming year. That is the word that is used—fix. All Methodist pastors are appointed every year. Either back to where they already serve, to a new appointment, or to retirement. Both Clara and I were on several conference committees, so our staff and church thought we would be out of town for the week, and I had already lined up a guest preacher for the 18th, so the church wasn't expecting to see us at the worship service.

Miraculously, without knowing anything in advance, Brandon and Emerson decided to cut their road trip short and come home early. I honestly believe Brandon "detected a disturbance in the force" and this contributed to him coming home early. He called me from West Virginia to tell me they would be home on Saturday, June 17th. I asked him to swing through Charlottesville on his way home (we lived in Yorktown, VA then) and pick up Taylor at UVa so the entire family could have dinner together. Emerson was going home to Dayton the next day, driving right through Charlottesville, so he could take Taylor back to school. I had gotten my wish. I was going to be able to tell all four children at the same time, which meant Clara and I were going to make an unexpected showing at church that Sunday, so we could tell the congregation. Brandon coming home when he did was a reminder to me that the Universe wasn't done with me yet, and I took it as a wink and a nod.

When your eighteen-year-old son goes on a fourteen-thousand-mile cross country trip, your prayer life gets full and enriching! I hadn't seen my son in three and a half months, and now he would be home on Saturday. Oh, the joy in my heart! He requested blackened yellow fin tuna with mango salsa (I am the chef in our family) for him and Emerson, and since it happened to be both Clara and Taylors favorite, I told him of course I would make it. In the kitchen prepping for dinner, I would suddenly and without warning just start weeping. I did that often in the early days. Trying to make sure neither Ryan nor Laura caught me weeping was a challenge. When I heard Brandon and Emerson pull up, I literally ran out the door and wrapped my arms around my sons, first the one that was gone so long, then the one away at school. I think I squeezed in a hug for Emerson as well. At least I hope I did. For one brief shining moment, all was right with my world. All of my children were home, and we were going to have a fabulous meal together.

My plan was to enjoy the meal, and afterwards tell them about me. But the kids quickly started talking about other friends who were either coming to our house after dinner, or where they wanted to go and I realized I had to do it *before* the meal. I don't remember exactly what I said, I just remember tears streaming down my face, and how all of them grew eerily quiet. Nobody said much during the meal mainly because no one knew what to say. Brandon had come home all excited to regale us with stories of his adventures, and I had taken that from him. That bothered me as much as what I had to tell them.

When considering my path ahead, I thought long and hard about refusing treatment. If I only had fourteen months to three years left to live, (an estimate given me during my first oncology appointment after diagnosis), did I really want to spend them going to doctor appointments, having my immune system beaten down by chemo, etc.? I talked to my nephew, Dr. Jason Moran, who was doing a fellowship in Boston at Beth Israel Deaconess Medical Center. He gave me some very sage advice. He let me know a new drug had just gotten approval that if I was able to take it, would allow me to be my own donor should I somehow make it to the point of a bone marrow transplant (or stem cell transplant. The two terms are interchangeable). He told me that new drugs and therapies were being discovered every day, and cautioned me, "What if something new comes out in a year or two that could wipe out your cancer, but you are too sick to take it?" He also reminded me of all the people who had gone before, who helped "move the needle" in relation to a cure for cancer. The last comment was what tipped the scales for me. I've always believed that when you get to a certain point in life it's time to turn around and give a hand up to those who are behind you. I decided to undergo chemotherapy with the goal of becoming eligible for a bone marrow transplant. That decision had already been made before I told my children.

As you might imagine, the dinner wasn't nearly as elegant as we had all hoped as we thought ahead to it. But we were all together. I said that night and many more times since, that I'm very glad this happened to me instead of to Clara or one of the kids. I was very sorry to drag them through all of this, but they understood it wasn't because of anything I did or did not do, and I knew they were behind me. It pained me that my announcement had to come the same day Brandon came home from his epic journey, but we had to get the word out, and I wanted to be in charge of the narrative.

The next day was Sunday, and the church we served, Saint Luke's United Methodist in Yorktown, VA had four worship services—at 8:30, 9:45, 11:00 a.m., and 5:05 p.m. I wanted everybody to hear the same thing, from me, even though I knew it would be all over the church after the 8:30 announcement. Remember, the church knew (thought) that Clara and I were at annual conference all the way across the state in Roanoke, Va. I texted my staff late the night before and asked them all to meet me in my office at 8 a.m. sharp, and to not speculate about the reason, especially with church members. As usual, my staff were all there just when I needed them to be. I am sure that most of them, like the church members, probably thought my meeting them at that time on that date meant the bishop had moved Clara and me at the 11th hour.

The meeting with the staff was very brief. Every one of them was stunned, many were in tears. I asked them to stay in my office until after the 8:30 service began, as church members seeing multiple staff members in tears would have prompted far more conversation than any of us were prepared for at that moment.

The 8:30 service began, and much to everyone's surprise, Clara and I walked out of the side door at the front of the sanctuary, holding hands and trying like hell to keep ourselves composed. We had agreed I would be the one to speak, so when we got to the front of the church, I did.

I don't remember exactly what I said, but it was along the lines of, "I know it comes as a shock to all of you to see Clara and I here in church when we are supposed to be at Annual Conference. To put your minds at ease, no, we are not moving." The congregation surprised me by applauding. I had to re-gather and re-center myself, as I was totally unprepared for that. But then I told them the reason why we were standing in front of them.

"I want you all to know that I have been diagnosed with Stage IVb mantle cell lymphoma, a very rare form of Non-Hodgkin lymphoma that has no known cause and no known cure. At this point I don't know what the future holds, I just know Who holds the future, so Clara and I ask for your prayers. But we also ask that you don't stop with us. (This was a request I was to make many, many times during the course of treatment). I am blessed with an amazing support structure, and I can assemble the best medical team in the world, and I want to state out loud that my intention is if one person in a million beats this it will be me. And remember, today is a GREAT day to be alive." You could have heard a pin drop as we walked out the door. I had to give that same Public Service Announcement three more times that day, and each time my initial comment about it not being about being moved was met with applause. That show of support even before the church knew what we were facing was and is an incredible source of manna for the journey for me.

In addition to telling our children prior to informing the church, we also told the Chair of our Staff Parish Relations Committee, Charlie Bates, and our District Superintendent, Seonyoung Kim. Both were incredibly moved and offered 100% support. I said this to the DS, "Please do not move me. We have lived here and ministered here going on 11 years, and this is where Clara and the children's friends and support structures are. Please don't take them away from that." Seonyoung is a quiet woman of deep faith and conviction who exudes a non-anxious presence. She assured me she would not allow me to be moved, and she kept her word. Thank you Seonyoung!

The next week I had a CT scan which showed lymphoma in 14 places in my body, including being above and below the diaphragm, in the gastrointestinal track and in my brain. Clara and I had my initial consult with Dr. John Kessler. He was compassionate, but realistic. I was facing some very long odds.

It was confirmed I was in Stage IVb and the five-year survival rate was nothing to write home about. But I was ready to begin the fight to evict the "Inglorious Bastard" that had invaded my body without my consent. (This is what I named the disease because I refused to give it the courtesy of calling it by it's name.) I told Clara, "When my time comes and I die, *Do Not* ever say that I 'lost my battle with cancer.'" If you are fighting cancer until the day you die, you have won! In the words of Winston Churchill—"When you are going through hell, keep going!"

For anyone reading this. If you or a loved one are battling cancer, when death comes, don't give cancer what it is not due. Don't put in an obituary that so and so "lost their battle with cancer." If you are fighting it until the day you die, you have won! Furthermore, during this battle you will come to the spiritual revelation, as Rumi said, that "the wound is the place where the Light enters you." I've also been shown that to understand the complexity of life and death, one must understand them as the same doorway. Death is part of life. All humans die. Death is never a battle to lose.

2

"The Most Difficult Thing is the Decision to Act, the Rest is Merely Tenacity."
~Amelia Earhart

Clara and I recently fell in love with a sitcom called, *The Kominsky Method*. During a recent episode one of the central characters said "when in doubt, ride the horse in the direction it's going." That quote pretty well sums up the start of treatment for me. One of the sobering and frightening things about a Stage IV diagnosis is the knowledge that when I am gone, life will go on. One of the comforting things about a Stage IV diagnosis is the realization that when I am gone, life will go on.

I had written out a bucket list of everything I wanted to do in the next eighteen months after my diagnosis, (like be present for my daughter's high school graduation and my son's graduation from college). I wrote down all the dates, and then working backward, figured out when my start date should be so I wouldn't miss any important date and I wouldn't mess up the chemo schedule. I began chemotherapy on July 14, 2016, which made everything work. It was two consecutive days every third week, with a projected first round of six to eight months. I also had an appointment scheduled to meet the Bone Marrow Transplant team at Virginia Commonwealth University Massey Cancer Center in Richmond, VA on July 19th.

The regime wasn't true chemotherapy. I was given a combination of Bendamustine and Rituxamab (B/R therapy). Rituxamab is a monoclonal antibody and only attacks lymphoma cells. In fact, it is so effective at killing them that I had to take a drug called Allopurinol for a week prior to starting it that would lower the uric acid in my body and help my kidneys eliminate the millions of dead cancer cells that were going to be lining up, awaiting disposal from my body. Bendamustine was the other drug. The World Health Organization has it on their list of essential medicines, which are medicines considered to be the safest and most effective. Trial results published in 2012 showed that using these two drugs in combination more than doubled disease progression-free survival rates. The B/R therapy also had significantly fewer side effects than older therapies.

The drugs are administered slowly, to see if your body can handle them. They start out at 50mg an hour and then increase the dosage until they figure out what your body can take. At one point during the first infusion my head start itching. I didn't think anything of it and asked Clara if she would scratch my head and neck. I'm like a little kid when it comes to having my head scratched. I'll pretty much promise you anything as long as you don't stop. Clara started scratching my head, then I asked her to scratch my neck and shoulders. Then I told her my tongue felt funny, at which point she said, "Don't you think you should tell them?" pointing to the nursing staff. Sure enough, I was having a full-blown reaction, but my pleasure in having my head scratched got in the way of any kind of judgment on my part as to what was happening. Thank God for our care-givers.

I was given a good size dose of steroids, and the reaction waned, but I was awake for the next thirty-six hours! We rejoiced in the knowledge that night was the first night in a very long time that I went to bed with fewer cancer cells in my body than when I woke up. As I lay sleepless in bed, I wondered about things such as—what was the precise moment when the lymphoma started? What was I doing? Who was I with? What was I thinking? These are unknowable questions, but when steroids keep you awake all night, your mind stays active.

On Friday July 1, Clara and two of our children, Taylor and Laura, attended a teaching session at Massey on how to handle things while I was receiving chemo. My immune system was being targeted by these drugs, and each time I received an infusion, my numbers would go lower, and my chance of infection would be higher. They learned how to properly clean the house, the sheets, the furniture, you name it! They also learned how to prepare my food; all meat had to be cooked to well-done, even though I preferred it medium rare, all produce had to be carefully washed—even the bananas. We could not accept any donations of food, which meant that as much as they wanted to, church members couldn't send over meals for me. We did find a loophole here, and people started sending over meals for the rest of the family, except for me. All my food had to be prepared in my own kitchen, and then, only by family members residing in the house. I was not allowed to clean up (not everything about cancer is bad), and I could not eat leftovers. This wasn't much of an issue for me, as I am notorious in my family for not eating leftovers. But now they learned, this was good sound medical advice!

I was allowed to continue to preach on Sunday mornings, but I had to wear a face mask during the service, except for when I was speaking. I was also not allowed to shake hands after the service, or greet people at the door on the way out. This was probably the hardest thing for me. After each service I would go to a little alcove behind the sanctuary, put my mask on and wait for the next service to begin. It really felt like a barrier between me and the people, and I didn't like it, but I abided by it. Those moments between each morning service became a time my Director of Music, Gordon Parr, and I would chat. The more time passed, the more I looked forward to and cherished these moments with Gordon. He became one of my chief confidants, and I knew whatever I said to him never went anywhere else.

Well-meaning and loving people would come up and ask me how I was doing. And while I appreciated their genuine care and concern, answering the same question several hundred times each Sunday was difficult. We started a "Caring Bridge" site, and asked people to go there to get the latest information on what was going on with me. Clara and I tried faithfully to keep this page updated, and it did cut down significantly on the repetitive questions. I am beyond humbled that as I write this, there have been over seventy-two thousand visitors to that site since we created it. You just go to the Caring Bridge website, enter the name of the person you're looking for, and if they have created a page, you can access it. Caring Bridge is free, open to anyone, and has other benefits such as a journal, a calendar and where you can request help.

As I was undergoing the B/R, we were also looking into other options. We were able to get an appointment with Dr. Gordon Ginder, Medical Director of MCV Massey Cancer Center. Traveling to Massey on July 13th, we hoped I would qualify for a nationwide clinical trial for lymphoma that he was coordinating. When we met with him, we found out the trial had been suspended indefinitely nation-wide, so that was out. But the good news Dr. Ginder shared with us was that the two yardsticks of measurement for lymphoma, known as MIPI and KI67 were both very low, which was great! These were explained to us as being like speedometers that measure the speed of the growth of the lymphoma cells. It meant the lymphoma was growing slowly and reproducing slowly, but it also suggested that it had been lurking in my body for quite a long time.

We started slowly settling in to what would be our "new normal." Every Tuesday morning was blood draw day. In my mind I likened it to an old show my parents played on the radio as we were having breakfast and getting ready for school. Callers into the radio station were asked if they knew "the count and the amount." If they got them both right—how many people had called in, and what the dollar total was, they won the money. I didn't *win* anything, but it was interesting to see where all my numbers went. The goal was to get me ready for a bone marrow transplant, which meant driving all my blood numbers as low as possible while still keeping me alive.

3

"Death is Not a Counterpoint or Contradiction to Life, but a Profound Teacher About the Meaning of Human Existence."
~Rabbi Abraham Joshua Herschel

"Human Beings can live without a lot of things, —except meaning" ~Viktor Frankl

This life/death balance reminded me of the above quote from Rabbi Abraham Joshua Herschel—I would continue to learn some very profound lessons about our life here on Earth.

As August began, I started having some severe side effects from the chemo. I started getting back pain that gradually worsened. I couldn't sleep for a couple of nights because there was no position where the pain was relieved. The only time I didn't feel the pain was during worship when I was preaching. Either my mind blocked it out, or I got a free pass from the Universe. Either way, preaching was a welcome relief.

I have always been willing to tackle issues from the pulpit. Sometimes to the consternation of church members who wished their political beliefs weren't in contrast to what the Gospel teaches and thus would prefer I not remind them of the dichotomy. But one thing cancer does is remove whatever vestigial filters a person may have had, and my preaching was as honest, transparent, direct and at times forceful as ever. I remember one week when I said to my congregation—"if you want to continue to believe the false narrative that "everything happens for a reason,' (it doesn't) then you are going to have to accept that one of those reasons is you are stupid." I remember pausing and looking out. I had their attention for sure! I continued. "If you step off a curb and get hit by a bus, is it divine providence—meant to be? Or did you just not look left? If you smoke two packs of cigarettes a day for thirty years and then develop cancer, is it 'all part of God's plan,' or are you just stupid?"

I was giving a sermon on "correcting bad theology." You know, phrases like, "Well, we must not question God." Or "everything happens for a reason." Neither of those statements are in the Bible, and neither of them are true. They are both a false narrative passed down through generations when we didn't know what else to say and felt obliged to say something. In the first church I served a young woman died of a brain aneurysm leaving behind a ten-year-old daughter. I had the difficult task of walking the young girl up to the casket when some well-meaning but theologically incorrect woman said to her, "Oh honey, you just have to accept this. God needed your mommy more than you do." I wanted to scream at the top of my lungs, "No HE doesn't! He has all the mommies He needs, and if He needs another one, He can make her out of a rib!"

But we humans shrink before the mystery of death and we come up with slogans to try and explain away the unexplainable.

Kate Bowler is a professor at Duke University, my alma mater, and wrote a book about her journey with Stage IV cancer entitled, *Everything Happens for a Reason And Other Lies I've Loved*. She does a wonderful job of debunking many of these "lies I learned in Sunday School." Things such as "everything happens for a reason." "God never gives you more than you can handle." Or the most insidious of all, "It's all part of God's plan." The community where I served for twelve years before taking medical leave and moving to Chesterfield, VA just experienced a tragedy on homecoming night. Three young men, all aged sixteen, were killed when the car they were in lost control, ran into a tree and flipped over. Try telling the parents of these young men that their son's death was "part of Gods plan!" Who would want to worship, serve, honor, or have anything to do with a God as callous as that?! No, their deaths were a tragic result of what happens when the laws of physics are not obeyed. Traveling too fast around a turn inevitably means you will lose control of your vehicle. God had no part in the planning or the execution of this event. God grieves with us and with our families, but God did not cause it or will it to happen. God will use this event to bring about good, but God did not orchestrate it for this purpose. Aside from teaching about what constitutes authentic versus inauthentic prayer, debunking some of these long held false beliefs is perhaps the hardest challenge in ministry.

I lost count of the number of people who theologically diagnosed my medical condition to me and who had no qualms sharing with me (or my wife, children, on social media etc.) their conclusions. At times I was told it was "so that I would inspire others" (if that was the case, why didn't God make me an Olympic champion?), it was so "God's greatness could shine," (doesn't it do that in a thousand other more tangible ways, like a sunset, or the changing leaves on a tree in the fall?). Of course, I was told that I was being punished for my sins and that I needed to repent. Like I said, my filters were gone, so I almost always asked the person "explaining" this last one to me why I got cancer and not them? A collage of their faces when I said this back to them would be hilarious. Despite my valiant efforts, I'm not sure I made much of a dent in the "everything happens for a reason, it's all part of God's plan" crowd. We cherish our slogans, our soundbites and our false beliefs even when the evidence against them is overwhelming.

Please, please resist the temptation to play armchair theologian or physician when someone you know has cancer. They are already getting hit with an overload of information, much of it new to them, and often in medical jargon that requires a translator. The last thing they need is for someone they know to prescribe some unproven, and more than likely harmful or even deadly treatment, just because you saw it on Facebook, or your cousin's friend neighbor tried it and is cured!

"You either get bitter or you get better. It's that simple. You either take what has been dealt to you and allow it to make you a better person, or you allow it to tear you down. The choice does not belong to fate. It belongs to you." ~Josh Shipp

I was not going to give in to the easy slogans to explain away my condition, nor was I going to allow myself to become bitter. I *was* going to get better!

The second B/R therapy was set to begin August 16, 2016. After battling severe pain, a bad case of hives and some other not as mentionable side effects during the first round, I was ready for round two.

Everything went smoothly. We were able to start out at a higher infusion rate as my maximum had been determined the first round, so it took much less time than before. However, my heart rate elevated and stayed elevated. We brought this to the attention of the nurses in the infusion room. First one put her stethoscope on me, said "hmmmm," and asked another to do it. Both of them asked a third and they told me I needed to come to another room and lie down while they performed an EKG on me.

It was somewhat of an ordeal as no one really knew how to hook up the portable machine they had. I don't think it had ever been used. Finally, Dr. Kessler came in, they attached it and sure enough, I was in Afib.

According to Heart.org, "Atrial fibrillation (Afib, or AF) is a quivering or irregular heartbeat (arrhythmia) that can lead to blood clots, stroke, heart failure and other heart-related complications. Normally, your heart contracts and relaxes to a regular beat. In Afib, the upper chambers of the heart (the atria) beat irregularly (quiver) instead of beating effectively to move blood into the ventricles. If a clot breaks off, enters the bloodstream and lodges in an artery leading to the brain, a stroke results. About 15–20 percent of people who have strokes have this heart arrhythmia. This clot risk is why patients with this condition are put on blood thinners."

Then the fun began. Dr. Kessler's office is right next door to Sentara Care Plex. In fact, coming in that morning I noticed a bright pink ambulance outside of it and remarked to Clara that it would be fun to ride in that. I would later be reminded to be careful what you wish/pray for.

Dr. Kessler said he thought it was crazy for me to wait the amount of time it would take to get an ambulance there, not to mention the cost, and suggested that two of the nurses just wheel me over there in a wheel chair. I am sure we looked like some kind of Keystone Cop routine as we ambled across the parking lot, and the attendant at the emergency room admitted that wasn't usually how people enter. It provided a moment of levity in an otherwise serious situation.

I was monitored in the emergency room for about three hours, and never went back into sinus rhythm (normal heart-beat), so I had to be transferred to the main hospital which had a cardiology unit. And guess how I was transported there? You guessed it, in the pink ambulance!

My heart rate stayed in the 120-140 range all afternoon and into the evening. I was surprised but not surprised when

Dr. Kessler showed up that evening to see how I was doing. I had been put in one room while awaiting an open bed in the cardiac unit, and one finally became available and I was moved. But he found me. As he was walking out the door I again said, "Thank you Dr. Kessler." He walked backward into my room just enough to be in it, look over at me and said, "Doug, its John," and left. What a wonderful person as well as a great doctor.

Like many other areas of our society, it has become more difficult to get in to a hospital to visit. This hospital took your picture and put it on a sticker along with the room number you were being allowed to visit. My daughter Laura and son Brandon came to visit me that night, and Laura forgot her ID. They let her in, but her sticker said she was the "possession of Brandon Gestwick." He loved that, she hated it! As our third and fourth children, they have always had a love/hate relationship, although as they have gotten older it has arced more to the loving side. One evening, years earlier, Laura was whining about some dinner item she didn't want to eat. Clara told her that there were only two pieces on her plate, so she had to eat one of them. Brandon promptly reached over quickly with his fork, stabbed the smaller piece and popped it into his mouth with a Cheshire Cat like grin, because now Laura had to eat the larger piece. Not only was she upset about that, but the laughs and giggles from the rest of the family made her none too happy. That one interaction explains a lot of the relationship between those two children. Brandon reveled in what her name tag said, while Laura hated it. As they were leaving, she tore it off, but it managed to come off in one piece. Brandon grabbed it from her but Clara got it from him and keeps it in the blue journal she carries with us to every appointment as she "scribes" for me.

The doctors were divided about my Afib. Some were of the mindset it was caused by chemo stress, others felt it might be genetic. My mother died of a stroke caused by Afib, and her brother, my uncle Homer has it as well. Regardless of origin, the decision was made to put me on a drug called Sotalol, which would be taken twice a day to regulate my heart rate and keep it in sinus rhythm.

According to the FDA—"To minimize the risk of induced arrhythmia, patients initiated or re-initiated on Sotalol hydrochloride tablets should be placed for a minimum of three days (on their maintenance dose) in a facility that can provide cardiac resuscitation and continuous electrocardiographic monitoring."

It was August sixteenth. My (our) wedding anniversary was August nineteenth, and at that point, I wasn't sure at all that this wasn't going to be the last anniversary we had together. I had already told Clara that I did not want to die in a hospital, and I sure didn't want to spend my wedding anniversary there! Especially if it might be the last one. The staff all got behind this goal (well, all but one, which I'll explain in a moment). The cardiologist came and said he felt it would be safe to discharge me after five doses. He explained he wanted to start it the morning of the seventeenth, not that evening, so a full complement of staff would be on hand if things went south. Two doses on the seventeenth, two on the eighteenth, and one the morning of the nineteenth, and I could get out of there.

That was the plan.

The morning of the nineteenth came and I was ready to get out of the hospital, forget about cancer and treatments and chemo and medicines just for a day and celebrate my wedding anniversary with my bride. But that morning, instead of my regular cardiologist, a Physician's Assistant whom I had never met came by for rounds. After she was through, I asked her what time I was being discharged, and she said it wouldn't be until the next day because I had to complete three full days of "loading." Loading is when you are started on a new medicine and are monitored continuously and watched carefully. I was taken aback and explained to her that my cardiologist told me he was going to discharge me after five doses, and I had just taken the fifth. She said that was nowhere in my chart so I asked her to call the cardiologist, who apparently did not work on Fridays. She said there was no need for her to call him, that she had made her decision and wasn't going to "take my word" that he had said I could be released after five doses. I then told her that she could discharge me, or I could disconnect all the tubes and monitors, but that one way or another, I was leaving the hospital that morning to celebrate my wedding anniversary. She snottily replied to me that if I left the hospital without being properly discharged, the insurance company wouldn't cover any part of the stay and I would be personally responsible for all the charges.

Like all dads, I have my repertoire of pithy sayings I roll out when it's to my advantage. One of them is this:

"The first thing you should know about me is that I'm not you. A lot more will make sense after that."

The other thing to know about me is I never back down from a challenge, and I never give up. Those qualities can admittedly be annoying at times, but have served me well throughout this entire journey, and no doubt have contributed to my still being alive. I don't ever take "no" for an answer, and will go over, around or if need be, THROUGH a wall if I feel I'm in the right. Once when Clara and I were having a marital spat, she put her hand on her hip and shook a finger at me with her other hand as she said, "You know the problem with you? The problem with you is you think you are always right."

I replied, "Well duh!"

She cocked her head and looked at me funny so I continued. "Of course I think I'm right. If I thought I was wrong, I'd think something different."

I thought I was right about not only wanting to get discharged to celebrate my anniversary, but also that my primary cardiologist had agreed to it, and I wasn't going to be stopped by this person's power play. And that was what I told her, that her power play was not going to stop me from celebrating my anniversary on what might be my last anniversary. Then I tried to appeal to her humanity. "Are you married?" I asked her

"Not exactly," she replied

"Not exactly?" I repeated. She then explained that it was really none of my business but she was separated from her husband and she had found out he was leaving her on their anniversary a few months earlier.

Now it all started making more sense. I said, "I'm not part of that drama, and I'm not paying the price for him." I asked her to leave and assured her I would be leaving the hospital that day, and felt no obligation to inform her as to when.

When we called the cardiology practice, we were informed that in fact *all* the cardiologists in the practice had gone to a continuing education event over the weekend and were unavailable. So I called Dr. Kessler and asked him if he could discharge me. "Of course," he said. He had been in the room when the cardiologist told me I could be released after five loading doses. He came over at lunchtime signed the orders, and I was free to go. Well, not exactly free. By hospital policy I had to be in a wheelchair to be transported out. The nurse who came to take me was none other than Nate DeHart, who had worked for me for five years as our Youth Director, before hiking the Appalachian Trail during which he clarified his call to nursing. He was a welcome face. As we were walking to the door, the PA passed us and then stopped. "I told you insurance wouldn't cover it if you just walked out of here!" She exclaimed loudly, for me and everyone in the hallway to hear.

"I'm not walking out, I got a ride." I said, making both Nate and Clara laugh.

"You have to be properly discharged." She said, running after us.

"He was," said Nate.

"By whom?' she asked

Nate looked at me and said loudly, "Just because she is violating all of your HIPPA rights by yelling your personal information in the hallway doesn't mean I'm going to."

So, I said, "John Kessler."

She looked a little puzzled and asked who was that.

"Dr. John Kessler, the physician that admitted me. It is OK with you if the admitting physician, a board certified and licensed oncologist with over thirty years of clinical practice discharges me, isn't it? I told you I didn't want any part of your power play, and that no matter what I would be discharged so I could celebrate my anniversary. And in addition to that, I will pray for you."

She didn't quite know what to make of that so turned on her heel, huffed and walked away. Nate helped me out of the wheelchair and into my car and we bid our goodbyes.

That night Clara and I celebrated our anniversary by driving over to Portsmouth, VA. It's only about a twenty-mile drive, but we had to traverse a river through a bridge-tunnel which made it feel a world away. Being on the other side of the tunnels again brought back a flood of memories. Our two oldest sons were born during the six years we were in Portsmouth. After dinner we drove past the hospital where they were born and reminisced. I was the pastor of Saint Mark in Churchland (fitting name) and Clara was the associate at Centenary, a few miles away. The first six years of our ministry was spent at these churches, and we were both ordained Elders in the United Methodist Church while we served here. I was taking a piano lesson from Clara's Music Director Everett Amos, when she came up behind me to tell me we were pregnant for the first time. We were both so excited. The book, What to Expect When You're Expecting, seemed as though it was written about us, and Clara had a textbook pregnancy. Everything went smoothly until delivery, and then the wheels fell off the bus. Clara was adamant that she didn't want to know the gender of our child until they were born. When the doctor came in to tell us that the baby was presenting posterior and was going into fetal distress and she was going to have to have an emergency Caesarean Section, we didn't know if he was talking about Ryan or Caitlin. (The names we had picked out if it was a boy or a girl). Clara was prepped and taken in for the procedure, and they allowed me to come in.

When Dr. Perwaiz started, he moved so fast that I know my eyes got as big as saucers. The nurse thought I was going to pass out from the blood, but I was just concerned that he had cut into my wife, very near my child, in less than a second. I remember thinking at the time that it should take him at least as long as it takes me to carve the Thanksgiving turkey!

The baby's head popped out through the incision, and they began to suction his nose. I said, "Gee Dad, you didn't tell me there was a side door. I've been trying to go out through the front door all night." Dr. Perwaiz let out a little chuckle, and without looking at me said, "You must not make me laugh, if you make me laugh you have to leave!" I made a motion across my face as though I was closing a zipper and didn't say another word. I still didn't know if I had a son or a daughter.

My father was an alcoholic who took his own life on Father's Day 1985, when I was just 28 years old. I didn't have a good relationship with him as I was growing up and especially not as I entered adulthood, and so without Clara knowing, I prayed every night of her pregnancy for a daughter. I didn't want to have a son and risk having the same relationship with him as I had with my father. But then they delivered the rest of our child, and as Ryan was pulled from his mother it was quite obvious, he was a boy. Which just goes to show that God answers all our prayers, He just doesn't always give us what we ask for! I'm actually extremely grateful that some things didn't work out the way I once wanted them to. Having not one but three sons, plus a daughter, are four of the biggest blessings in my life. My marriage to Clara makes five—I would not change a thing.

At our first visit with Dr. Perwaiz following Ryan's birth, after we had gone over all the medical stuff Dr. Perwaiz said he wanted to talk to us. He told us that he had never been married, choosing instead to be a one-person gynecological office, but that if he ever did marry, he would want to have a relationship like we had (I'm 100% sure he never saw us at our worst moments!) and he wanted to give us a gift. He told us that he was refunding every dollar we had paid him so far, and would not charge us anything in the future and hoped we would stay with him for future children. What an amazing and unexpected gift.

We had a great deal of difficulty conceiving a second child, and month after month we were heart broken when Clara was still not pregnant. But it finally happened when Ryan was almost two and a half. Taylor was due April fourth, but came on the first. I had to tell everyone I called with the news that no, it was not an April Fool's joke, our child had been born. As we did with Ryan, we did not find out Taylor's gender until he was born. But what was different was the delivery. Clara long lamented that she was knocked out for Ryan's birth and didn't get to experience it, and she was bound and determined to give birth "naturally." A vaginal birth after Caesarean (VBAC) is not common, but it is doable in some situations. Dr. Perwaiz was firmly behind it and this time the labor progressed as it should. When the baby's head crowned, Dr. Perwaiz turned to me and said, "I'll be the coach, you be the quarterback." I wasn't exactly sure what he meant until he asked me, "Would you like to deliver your own child?"

I was flabbergasted and in tears, but said yes. I scrubbed and gowned up, and he stood behind me and coached me the whole way through, and my hands were the very first hands to ever touch Taylor in this world. That was a life moment I will never ever forget. "Taylor Williams Gestwick, welcome to the world," I said as I kissed his head. Clara was fully awake and present for this birth so I handed him to his mother.

As we were having our children, deciding on names was always a challenge. We would each make lists, then swap them with each other and cross a certain number off. We really couldn't come to agreement.

We had talked to my mother about this and the names we were considering, Taylor being one of them when she said, "Oh, Taylor Williams, that was my grandfather's name." We had already settled on the name Amanda if the baby was a girl.

Not long after he was born, my mother sent Taylor a long, handwritten letter where she shared with him all her remembrances of her grandfather, and she even included a picture of him, with his cousin—Amelia Earhart.

I immediately called my mother.

"Mom, we're related to Amelia Earhart?! How come you never told me? All those biographies I had to write in high school, and I never knew this?!"

Her response was, "Well, you never asked"

I said, "Hitler, Mussolini, c'mon Mom, this isn't information you should hold back from your kids!"

Years later when I got heavily in to doing genealogy, I discovered that we were in fact, related to Amelia Earhart, but she was my seventh cousin, twice removed. While our families probably never had Thanksgiving dinner together or exchanged presents at Christmas it was still pretty cool.

As Clara and I drove home from our anniversary dinner, we shared reminiscences of our first parsonage and where our first two children had been born. When we lived there, we had planted two trees in the backyard and one in the side yard, and the massive size of the trees astounded us. It was incredible to see how much they had grown. As we headed back home that night, I told Clara how wonderful it was that we had gotten lost in the moment and the memories, and that for the last hour, I didn't think at all about cancer, or dying, or leaving my wife and children behind. I remember something I had seen on Facebook:

> "If you focus on the hurt, you will continue to suffer,
> If you focus on the lesson, you will continue to grow."

I was bound and determined more than ever to focus on the lesson. Our twenty-seventh anniversary was one of the best we ever celebrated, and reminded me of how much I had to live for, and how much the fight was worth it.

One of my staff members at Saint Luke's, James Pace, was diagnosed with leukemia on his 49th birthday, and died a few days before his 50th birthday. His illness taught Saint Luke's how to deal with a senior staff member facing a life-threatening illness, and graced us in innumerable ways. His wife, Rachel, wrote on my Caring Bridge site on August 27th, 2016:

"The only time I saw James cry during his illness was when we had to tell our daughter Emily that he was dying. He had tried so hard to protect her. The instinct to protect those we love is so strong. And as someone who was on the other side of it, what hurt me the most was seeing his pain and not having the power to fix it. But, looking back, I am grateful for the opportunity to have gone through that time with him. You never really know how much you love someone until you learn to hold each other up in the hardest times. Regardless of the outcome, I was given a gift in that love." Rachel is a gifted writer and I hope some day every one who reads this book and more will be exposed to how she captures the essence of life in the written word.

Most people shy away from conversations about death. But they are some of the deepest, most meaningful discussions you can have in life. On the day of my birth, my death began its walk. It is walking toward me, without hurrying. One day we will meet. I am doing everything I can to delay that day. That I can do. But what I cannot do is to stop it. Talking about death with loved ones is one of the most sacred and profound conversations you can have. What I used to shun I now cherish.

4

Being Alone Has a Power Very Few People Can Handle.

Only those who care about you can hear you when you're quiet.

On August 30th I made a Caring Bridge entry telling everyone that my white blood count was so low that I could no longer interact with anyone other than my immediate family. I was still going to my office at the church, but asked everyone to stop at my door and not come in. I also wore a face mask during worship and only took it off when I was preaching. This was so very hard on me. I felt like more and more walls were being built between me and everyone else, but I also couldn't risk any kind of infection.

On August 31, 2016, Clara and I had one of the hardest meetings we were to have throughout this whole journey. We met with the director of Pension and Benefits for the Virginia Annual Conference, John Fuller, and the benefits administrator, Nancy Blair. I had served eight years on the Conference Pensions and Benefits Committee and knew both of them very well. This meeting was to discuss all the benefits Clara would have when I died. It was an emotional meeting from the start, as I had to say, "when I die" and "when I am gone" far too often during the meeting. Nancy and John were as emotionally engaged as Clara and I were, and they too shed numerous tears. We reviewed in detail the conference health insurance benefits, and how to maximize what is covered and what changes when I die and am no longer the primary insured. We drafted a plan for how she and the kids would be covered after my death. We went over all the various United Methodist pension plans and what she should do to maximize the benefits from mine. We reviewed our long-term care insurance and what had to happen for that to kick in. We reviewed the denominations relationship with Ernst and Young and the way for her to receive their advice. I cannot say "thank you" enough to John Fuller and Nancy Blair. They are simply the best. I've spent my entire adult life making sure my wife and children would be taken care of in the event something happened to me. And now it was. The meeting with John and Nancy was hard, there is no other way to describe it. *So* many tears were shed. But they both hung in there with us, and shared not only our tears, but their expertise, and I left feeling very confident that my dear darling bride and our four beautiful children would be well taken care of when I died.

We were approaching the third round of B/R therapy, and my blood numbers were all very low. This was the goal, but the practical result was I was exhausted all the time, and very susceptible to infection. My sister Diane and her husband Charlie came to visit and buoyed my spirits. I told them that if I had known that getting cancer would mean all my siblings came to visit me in Virginia, I would have gotten it years earlier!

I wrote on my Caring Bridge site that the old saw about "what doesn't kill you makes you stronger" was a lie. The Mantle Cell lymphoma and its treatment made me weaker, much weaker, but I was determined that no matter what, every single day when my feet hit the ground I would exclaim, "It's a great day to be alive!" and believe it.

On September 13th Clara and I met with my oncologist, Dr. John Kessler, and he was really thrilled with the progress I had made. We scheduled some additional tests to see where I was overall, but things were starting to look like I would be able to apply for a bone marrow transplant, something we didn't even know how to dream about when this journey first began.

Life started to take on a new rhythm. Every Tuesday was still blood draw day. The third B/R therapy I had was the easiest one ever, and for once, there were no complications during the infusion. The fatigue and nausea for a few days after was becoming part of my new normal. I told a friend of mine there is an "incredible lightness of being" that comes with a terminal diagnosis. There is just a clarity about life that perhaps can come no other way. Maybe it's God's or The Universe's way of giving back something to those who find themselves with my draw in life. I'm taking this as a gift. I never anticipated this or thought it would be my lot. But here I am. And I have been given a gift few achieve. I have a clarity of consciousness about life that is unique and laser-focused. And it is very hard to put into words. The Bible says in Romans 8:26 that the Holy Spirit intercedes with "sighs too deep for words." I completely understand that now. The lightness of being is an incredible, relief filled, deep-breathed knowledge that all will be OK. I am going to take a step into eternity before the others who I love so deeply it cannot be measured, *but*, that step will not take me away from them, it will bring them closer to me. Cancer teaches you to be in tune with your own body in ways that one would never learn if they did not have it. Honestly, yes, I would prefer that I was out of tune here, but I'll take the Grace cancer gives even if I didn't select it as my teacher. Paul Tripp once wrote,

"Waiting is not just about what I get at the end of the wait, but about who I become as I wait."

As the senior pastor of a very large, multi-staff church for many years I learned that whatever I focused on grew. If I focused on a problem, it grew. If I focused on a solution, it grew. I used to joke with my colleagues that we had to be careful because being a senior pastor was a lot like being a Basilisk. Repetitive complaining will attract things for you to complain about. Repetitive gratitude will attract things for you to be thankful about. I was becoming a more grateful, patient and loving husband, father and person, and for that I gave thanks.

"Sometime you must hurt in order to know, fall in
order to grow, lose in order to gain, because most
of life's greatest lessons are learned through pain"
~Masashi Kishimoto

C.S. Lewis, that great Christian novelist and theologian wrote, "Hardships often prepare ordinary people for an extraordinary destiny."

On my Caring Bridge site on September 28, I posted a poem that has meant a lot to me over the years. I first came across it as an undergraduate in the 1970's, and at various points in my life I have gone back to it. It's titled The Desiderata. In some places it is attributed to Max Erhman in 1927, others places say it was found in Old Saint Paul's Cathedral in 1692. Either way, there is no copyright on it, so I'll share it here as well:

Go placidly amid the noise and the haste, and
remember what peace there may be in silence.
As far as possible, without surrender, be on good terms
with all persons.
Speak your truth quietly and clearly; and listen to
others, even to the dull and the ignorant; they too have
their story.
Avoid loud and aggressive persons; they are vexations
to the spirit.
If you compare yourself with others, you may become
vain or bitter, for always there will be greater and lesser
persons than yourself.

Enjoy your achievements as well as your plans.

Keep interested in your own career, however humble; it is a real possession in the changing fortunes of time.

Exercise caution in your business affairs, for the world is full of trickery.

But let this not blind you to what virtue there is; many persons strive for high ideals, and everywhere life is full of heroism.

Be yourself. Especially do not feign affection. Neither be cynical about love; for in the face of all aridity and disenchantment it is as perennial as the grass.

Take kindly the counsel of the years, gracefully surrendering the things of youth.

Nurture strength of spirit to shield you in sudden misfortune.

But do not distress yourself with dark imaginings. Many fears are born of fatigue and loneliness.

Beyond a wholesome discipline, be gentle with yourself. You are a child of the universe no less than the trees and the stars; you have a right to be here. And whether or not it is clear to you, no doubt the universe is unfolding as it should.

Therefore be at peace with God, whatever you conceive Him to be.

And whatever your labors and aspirations, in the noisy confusion of life, keep peace in your soul.

With all its sham, drudgery and broken dreams, it is still a beautiful world.

Be cheerful. Strive to be happy.

In late September 2016, Clara and I took a week's vacation and drove up the east coast to Boston, and then on to New Hampshire. My nephew Jason was the chief resident of Brigham and

Women's Hospital, and was doing a fellowship in immunology and oncology. He had been so helpful to both Clara and I throughout this journey, so we took him and his wife Christina out to a fancy dinner at a wonderful restaurant in Back Bay. My best friend Bruce Jones also joined us. When I stepped away from the table, Jason asked Clara how she was doing. She replied, "I have lost my ability to dream. I can't imagine a tomorrow because I don't know if Doug will be there." Jason's reply to her was encouraging. He said, "Doug is going to live a long life." Thank you, Jason! That encouragement was powerful medicine for Clara's soul.

After dinner we traveled with Bruce to his home in New Hampshire. All the clergy benefit plans in the United Methodist Church are underwritten by Liberty Mutual Insurance Company, and Bruce was the head actuary there. I brought along a copy of the benefit notebook Clara and I had earlier gone over with John Fuller and Nancy Blair, and explained it all to Bruce, and he explained it all to me. I told him that when I die, I've told Clara she should lean on him, and take his advice when it came to these benefit plans. I was also able to cross off another item on my bucket list. On my original list I had written "cook for Bruce and Kellie in New Hampshire." Now I was able to. We had a wonderful visit, great food and wine and conversation. Just what the doctor ordered.

The first week of October came and my church, Saint Luke's, was a remote host for our Conference Five Talent Academy. Our Bishop, Sharma Lewis, was preaching, and I felt like she was speaking directly to me. She started out by saying Faith is an action, while Fear is a reaction. That resonated deeply with me. She then went on to make three important points about faith.

Faith is:
Believing when you don't see

**Obeying when you don't understand, and
Persisting when you feel like giving up.**

Talk about food for the journey! Bishop Lewis gave me this life-giving sustenance, that, like manna, came just when I needed it and in exactly the right amount.

The following week was going to be a big one for me. I had my fourth round of B/R therapy and then was scheduled to go to Richmond and meet with the Stem Cell transplant team at Massey Cancer Center. I told Clara that I was going to believe even if I don't see it, obey even when I don't understand, and persist if I ever feel like giving up. One thing I've learned in life is that the difference between success and failure is that one extra time you muster the strength to rise. That week I wrote in my journal—"One day, the mountain that is in front of you will be so far behind you, it will barely be visible in the distance. But the person you become in learning to get over it? That will stay with you forever. And that is the point of the mountain."

We went to Dr. Kessler's office where we had an appointment with him prior to having round four B/R therapy. He gave us some startling news. I had reached "NED." There was one anomaly though. Thirteen of the original fourteen "lights" in my body had gone out. (Areas "light up" indicating areas of metabolic activity. Not always, but frequently these are areas of concern). One, in my right lung, had not only stayed, but it also grew in size. It was very small, less than 5cm, but it had stayed and grown so it was something we had to watch. The blood flow cytometry also came back negative, meaning it could not detect any lymphoma in my blood.

NED stands for "No Evidence of Disease." It is the goal of all cancer treatment, and I had to get to this stage to even be considered for a bone marrow, or stem cell transplant.

Dr. Kessler explained it like this:

"When you look out your window and see all sorts of weeds in your lawn, you decide to do something about it. You go out and buy a bunch of weed killers and spread them on your lawn. Soon, all the weeds are gone. Or so it appears. This is No Evidence of Disease. *But,* lurking under the soil are seeds and roots which if left untreated will come back as weeds. To really get rid of the weeds for good, you let the grass go to seed, which you collect. Then you tear out the entire turf, and put down some even more powerful herbicides, ones that will destroy the roots and seeds and everything else. Then you replant the weedless seed you collected, and now your lawn is truly 100% weed free, not just one that looks like it."

The B/R therapy was doing its job. We were going to keep an eye on the one spot in my lung that stayed on and do some additional testing, but I had reached the first step towards qualifying for a stem cell transplant.

There had been some question about whether I would ever get to NED, given that I started out as advanced Stage IV. To get there after only three rounds of B/R therapy, with another three scheduled was amazing. Clara and I once again cried really hard with each other, but they were now tears of joy, not sorrow.

That troublesome spot in my right lung did not go away with the B/R therapy. So what was it? No one knew for sure. The only way to find out was to have a procedure called a Navigational Bronchoscopy. This involves going in to my lung with a special scope, guided by a live CT feed. Once at the site, the doctor would do a series of procedures to collect samples so pathology could determine what it was. It could be lymphoma, or another type of cancer, or it could be an infection of some kind. Whatever it was, we had to get rid of it before the transplant, or I would not be allowed to undergo it. There was one small problem, however. As it was explained to us, our insurance company, Anthem Blue Cross/Blue Shield, was the ONLY insurance company on the face of the planet that did not cover this procedure. Even though its effectiveness had been proven in study after study, Anthem BC/BS still considered it "experimental" and would not cover it. Our conference benefits officer tried talking to the insurance company. "No." The pulmonologist who was going to do the procedure tried talking to the insurance company. "No." We were not able to make any headway. With all the other medical bills that were piling up, there was not any way I could afford to pay for this procedure out of pocket, particularly when none of the payment would go towards my yearly deductible. Between the doctor, hospital, anesthesiologist etc., the amount was close to $30,000. Clara kept urging me to go ahead with it, but I balked. I was determined to not bankrupt my family through this illness. The money we had put away for retirement was to support us (her) for the rest of our lives. I wasn't going to withdraw it, pay an early withdrawal penalty *and* pay taxes on it, for a procedure with an uncertain outcome.

Clara and I literally fought over this issue. She kept saying she didn't care about the money. She would rather work every day for the rest of her life than have the money we saved from *not* doing the procedure, and live knowing that decision resulted in my death.

It was a very stressful time, and obvious that neither of us were going to budge from our position.

We went back in to see the pulmonologist, Dr. Todd Duggan, who made us the proverbial offer you can't refuse. He said he would be willing to forgo all of his fee if the hospital was willing to do the same. His head nurse got on the phone with someone at the hospital, and they agreed that this situation was life-threatening for me, and that if Dr. Duggan was willing to do it pro bono, they were too.

We certainly did not expect this at all, and his generous offer reduced both of us to tears. He said that he made plenty of money, that he didn't get in to medicine to make money, he got into medicine to save lives, and he also thought that perhaps they might be able to get Anthem BC/BS to change their policy if they could demonstrate the effectiveness of this procedure. True to his word, Dr. Duggan did not bill me for the procedure, although it took many months, phone calls, emails and personal visits for the hospital to make good on their side.

During one visit with him, I noticed he was writing in my chart with his left hand. Clara, Taylor and Brandon are all left-handed in our family. When we would go out to dinner as a family right-handers sat on one side of the table, left-handers on the other. I told Dr. Duggan that Clara had a tee-shirt that said "Everyone is born left-handed, you turn right-handed after you commit your first sin." He nodded and murmured something and about ten seconds later without saying a word or looking up, he deftly switched the pen into his right hand and kept writing. It cracked me up on a day when laughter was greatly needed.

I had the navigational bronchoscopy. If you think of your lungs as trees, you can visualize what was going on. Thick wide airways branch off into smaller ones, which in turn branch off into even smaller ones, which themselves branch off even smaller. The object was so tiny, and off one of the very smallest branches, and really hard to reach. Dr. Duggan thought he got a piece of it but was not 100% sure. We waited for the pathology reports to come back still not knowing what it was.

In the meantime, we had a few other challenges or setbacks, or whatever you want to call them. I like to refer to them as FGE, but that is not very pastoral, so I leave it to you the reader to decipher what I mean by that.

Clara and I met in 1987 when she began seminary at Duke. The year prior, her father had experienced a heart attack. He had been on a long, slow yet steady decline ever since I knew him. From that first year, every Thanksgiving we would celebrate with her family. Once the grandchildren appeared, we added a Christmas celebration on Thanksgiving weekend and nicknamed it "Thankxmas." For about ten years every time we were on the way home from Thankxmas invariably one of us would ask the other, "Do you think this is the last time we will see Pepop?" Pepop was the name given to her father by our oldest son Ryan, who was also the oldest grandchild. And it had stuck. Everybody called him Pepop—even Clara's mother when she was alive. When I first got diagnosed, I promised Clara that I would outlive Pepop. Several times along the journey I questioned whether I could do that, but it seemed like a safe bet at the time. And in the end, I did outlive my father-in-law.

This time when she went to see him, she got rear ended at a traffic light. No real serious damage, but I think it was just the straw that broke the camel's back for Clara. She had been under so much stress, both because of my situation and her father's deteriorating health, that this was what did her in. She sobbed uncontrollably on the phone, and I just let her. Sometimes a good cry is the most cleansing tonic in the world.

While she was in South Carolina our son Brandon called me. Brandon never just chit chats on a phone call. He always jumps right to the point. One evening when he was in middle school, he called from summer church camp. I was pleased to see his number pop up and I answered, "Hey Brandon." Before I could say anything else he blurted out, "When did I have my last tetanus shot?" Not the first line you want to hear from your child away at camp, but that's Brandon.

On this call the first thing he said was, "Do you know that your truck is not registered in the State of Virginia?" I had a

2001 Ford F-150 and this was 2016. It had been registered in Virginia for fifteen years. "What in the world are you talking about? Of course its registered." He put the police officer on who explained the situation to me. Brandon and a couple of friends had taken an old john boat they had repurposed and launched it off the Colonial Parkway near Williamsburg—a definite no-no! This officer saw them, and when he talked to them, it was obvious they had no idea they were doing anything wrong. He also noticed that my registration was out of date. The State of Virginia sends renewal notices by email, and I looked back and found the one they sent me—which had come the day after I was diagnosed with cancer. I never saw it because I never opened it. He said that with the multiple violations he had to give Brandon a ticket for something, and the registration was the least expensive and wouldn't cost him any points on his license. I explained my situation and all I was dealing with and begged the officer to issue it to me and not Brandon since I was the one at fault, but to no avail. Ultimately when Brandon went to court for the ticket the judge just dismissed it, so all turned out well.

We got notice from Anthem BC/BS that they had denied the claim for my navigational bronchoscopy, which we anticipated. However, the same week we got a notice from our car insurance company that they mistakenly dropped two major discounts we were entitled to. Because our account was set up on auto pay, we got charged a much higher amount than we owed. But not to worry, they told me, it would be refunded in two to three business cycles, meaning months. I called and kept calling and kept going up the corporate ladder, letting State Farm know I really wasn't happy with them issuing themselves a short-term interest free loan from my checking account, but of course my appeal fell on deaf ears. Verizon wireless did the same to us. They charged us full retail price for Brandon upgrading his phone to a new iPhone 7 and for making long distance calls to Canada. Only problem was, he did neither! Apparently a "glitch" in Verizon's system caused the 1.2 million people who were within a month of being able to upgrade their equipment to be charged as though they had. They assured us though, the $65 loan they had reached into my bank account and given themselves would be refunded in November.

Normally I would take things like this in stride and just keep working my way up the phone ladder until I got someone who realized it was in their corporate best interest to help me immediately, not refund me six to eight weeks later. But with everything else going on, and not sure what was going on with my lungs, these two things gave me an outlet to focus my anger and angst, and boy did I! When I was talking to the Verizon vice-president, I did the math for her and said "1.2 million people X $65 is $78 MILLION dollars that Verizon has "inadvertently" loaned themselves, interest free, out of their customers bank accounts." This is not insignificant.

Fighting these battles let me forget for a time that something was growing in my right lung and we didn't know what it was.

We finally got the initial report back from the bronchoscopy which indicated it was *not* cancer or infection. While we rejoiced in this news, there was a big part of me that was very skeptical. "If it's not cancer or infection, then what *is* it?" I wondered during the many sleepless nights that followed. Clara was happy with the report, and with all she had on her plate being my primary caregiver and wife, I wasn't about to voice my concerns to her. I was sure that somehow whatever it was would be found out soon enough, and if she could have some days of joy and relief, I wasn't going to take those from her.

On November 1, 2016, I had my normal Tuesday morning blood draw at VOA (Virginia Oncology Associates). It was kind of weird to see the door open and a female nurse call my name and *she* had a mustache. But when I got back in the lab, *all* the nurses had some form of facial hair. "No shave November" started out as "Movember," a time when men would grow out their mustaches in support of fund raisers for all men's cancers. That morphed into No Shave November. I remember when my boys started doing this in high school. I thought it was just an excuse to be scruffy and not shave, but it's a real thing.

The week before my brother Dan had called me and said he and his son Evan were talking about doing "No Shave November" in my honor and asked if my boys would participate too. I told him I would and I was sure they would too. When they heard about the challenge, both my wife Clara and my daughter Laura also offered to participate, an offer I politely declined.

Dan wanted to publicize it, and set up a Go Fund Me site to help me pay my medical bills. I was reluctant at first, because I never ever want to ask someone for something, especially not church members. I told him he could set it up and publicize it all he wanted, but that I did not want it publicized through Saint Luke's. So many other people were dealing with things in their life equally as difficult as my situation, and I didn't feel right benefiting financially from my position as senior pastor. In the end, a few individuals and groups from the congregation of Saint Luke's did contribute, but we were able to keep it from being a distraction within the church.

To say I am/was grateful doesn't even begin to scratch the surface of my feelings. Cancer is expensive. I don't know how people without quality health insurance manage it, but I know I couldn't. I had great insurance but I still had thousands of dollars in out-of-pocket costs, copays, and a potential *huge* bill from the hospital for the bronchoscopy. This fund raiser my brother put together came at the exact right time in my life, and allowed me the freedom to exhale, to breathe in deeply, to not worry about finances and just focus on healing. Thank you, Dan. Love you brother!

Meanwhile, the B/R therapy was doing what it was supposed to do, which was to drive my blood numbers low, but not too low. I was exhausted all the time. I remember several times when I was playing cello that I would fall asleep and wake up thirty or forty minutes later, still holding my bow and cello. Thankfully I didn't damage either one.

We were progressing towards a stem cell transplant after the first of the year. In addition to our family tradition of "Thankxmas," November was also the time I would take an annual hunting trip. I would go to Bergton, VA the week before Thanksgiving to hunt with my dear friends Dewey Swicegood and Neal Snoddy, and then I would travel to South Carolina where I would hunt with the Price family, my boys, and anyone else who came. These were such cherished days and memories in my life, and I was thankful I was going to be able to do it again. However, Clara wasn't willing to just let me go off into the woods with a gun and a knife, so she sent our youngest son Brandon along with me to Bergton. Brandon had been my "hunting buddy" more than any of my other children, and often said that hunting together in South Carolina will always be his best memory of our time spent together. The week of Thanksgiving was the first week since June that I did not have *any* doctor appointments or procedures or scans or anything scheduled. Unless you've experienced this you have no idea how amazing it is to get a "get out of jail free" card like this!

At Bergton, Brandon hit it off with Dewey and Neal much as I had. We were skinning a very small deer I had shot, and Dewey and Neal were giving me a hard time, as guys often do. Brandon enjoyed that so much he exclaimed, "Man, you guys are so great, I just wish you were younger." We all got a hearty laugh out of that, but in that moment, Brandon became "one of us," and has been on the Bergton hunt every year since. I told Neal and Dewey that when I was gone, I hoped they would invite Brandon for the annual hunt, and they assured me they definitely would.

As the year ended, I had my final B/R infusion in December, and we were actively working towards scheduling the stem cell transplant. I had a PET scan on December 1 and then Clara and I went to Massey to have as much of the pre-op work done as possible. Since we had met all the insurance deductibles and out of pocket maximums, we were trying to schedule as much as we could before the end of the year.

The PET scan results came back, and that troublesome spot in my right lung still lit up. The only problem was, we still didn't know what it was. It could be another cancer; it could be an infection. Whatever it was, it was "taking up" in the scans. "Taking up" is when an area absorbs the dye or contrast they are using and is indicative of some malady.

My blood numbers continued to drop, which is what we wanted. The last infusion brought on an unbelievable increase in nausea and exhaustion. My hemoglobin and hematocrit numbers were so low I was basically anemic. My white blood count was also extremely low, which left me susceptible to infection easily.

I read a quote from Jim Kelly, the hall of fame quarterback from the Buffalo Bills (my hometown) that really resonated with me. Jim has fought his own battle with insidious cancer, and its return, and has done so very publicly and very courageously. He said, "Go make a difference today for someone who is fighting for their tomorrow." In addition to, "It's a great day to be alive," I added this to my sign off on Caring Bridge.

My last B/R infusion was on December 6. My white blood count was under the minimum needed to do the infusion, but after consultation with my doctor, Dr. John Kessler, I decided to go ahead and have it anyway. I had to sign a waiver of liability, which I gladly did. *Nothing* was going to stop me from getting to the stem cell transplant!

Every year during the Advent season, Saint Luke's has a church wide Advent dinner celebration. This is a church of almost 2000 members, and in one night we *all* have dinner together. It is quite a logistical undertaking. And every year the Music Director, Gordon Parr, brings his Tabb Girls Ensemble (Tabb is one of the high schools served by Saint Luke's) for a concert. I could not sit in the sanctuary like I normally would, because there were too many brand-new germs brought in. I sat out in the Narthex (a funny church word to describe any space adjacent to the sanctuary). Towards the end of the concert, Gordon stood up and asked me to come in. As I walked up to the front, Gordon's voice began to break, and he told the assembled crowd his take on everything I had gone through. He then said his choir had learned a special piece and he wanted them to do it in my honor. It was, "In the Arms of An Oak" by Andy Beck. If you Google it, you will find it says, "This special piece is a loving tribute to those who stand strong throughout life's seasons and storms." Gordon and his choir had me in tears, and I did something I hadn't done in months and wasn't supposed to do. I hugged him.

President Roosevelt described December 7 as "a day that will live in infamy." It was for me, and not because of Pearl Harbor. December 7, 2016 was the last infusion of B/R. Six months earlier when I had been diagnosed with Stage IVb lymphoma I didn't even know if I would live to see this day. Now here it was, I had completed the first segment of treatment successfully and I was looking ahead to a stem cell transplant. After my port was flushed, I got to take part in a ritual at Virginia Oncology Associates and rang a cow bell. The rest of the patients and staff all cheered and clapped, and I got my picture taken under a big sign that said, "Today you are a survivor."

Christmas came early for me. As I reflected on my journey, I thought that whenever someone in the church dies, we say they have "claimed the promise of the resurrection." As I moved through Advent,

I realized that before we claim the promise of the resurrection, we need to claim the promise of the Incarnation. Emmanuel. God with us.

When I rang the cowbell at Virginia Oncology Associates, I was claiming the promise of the Incarnation. Emmanuel. God with me.

5

"Sometimes the Fear Does Not Subside and One Must Choose to do it Afraid."
~Elisabeth Elliott

"Let me tell you something you already know. I don't care how tough you are. You, me or nobody gonna hit as hard as life. But it aint about how hard ya hit. It's about how hard you can get hit and keep moving forward. How much you can take and keep moving forward. That's how winning is done."
~Rocky Balboa

On December 9th, I wrote the following in my Caring Bridge journal—"Life had hit me and my family pretty hard since June. Each round of chemo knocked me down hard and harder than the one before it. But I got up each time, and I am going to continue to get up. I will never give up; I will always get up. I don't care how hard I get hit, and by all accounts the stem cell transplant is going to hit me harder than anything before it. But I am going to get up. I will NEVER give up. I am going to beat this inglorious bastard that has invaded my body. I'll take every shot it throws at me and I will keep moving forward. That's how winning is done. I refuse to lose."

Reading back over it, I can see I was writing that to myself as much as I was to anybody else. The difference between failure and success is that one extra time you find the strength to rise.

The B/R regime had done its job. It got me to and past

the NED stage. My white blood count was less than one third of what the low end should be. My neutrophils (neutrophils make up most of your white blood count and are crucial in fighting infections) were well below half the minimum number and all my red cell counts were below minimums. I had to stay away from everybody but my immediate family. It was hard to be cocooned upstairs in our bedroom, especially during the Christmas Season. Brianna Weist wrote—

> "One day, the mountain that is in front of you will be so far behind you, it will barely be visible in the distance. But the person you become in learning to get over it? That will stay with you forever. And that is the point of the mountain."

I was certainly facing a mountain. I wasn't sure where the journey was going to take me, but I was bound and determined to have more time in this life with my wife and family. During the darkest days and roughest parts ahead, that thought is what sustained me.

We were on the pre-transplant stage of test after test after test. I had pulmonary function tests, a bone marrow biopsy, and a "first pass" nuclear scan in the cardiac wing, along with one-on-one meetings with each of the key doctors and technicians involved with the stem cell transplant. A bone marrow transplant, or stem cell transplant, is one of the most brutal procedures you can put your body through. Literally they kill you (or come awfully close to it) to bring you back to life. My deeper concern was for Clara and the kids. I was confident I could handle anything life threw at me, but it pained me to the depths of my soul to see the hurt and uncertainty they were going through. I remember when I was a little child my mother would often say to me, "You just don't know when to quit." When she said it to me, it wasn't a compliment. But I was going to prove her right. I wasn't going to quit, no matter what!

Where we lived in Yorktown was about a ninety-minute drive to Massey. When I would have a five-minute scan, it was an hour and a half there, and an hour and a half back. Clara and I used these rides to deepen and strengthen our relationship. We talked about the kids, and what we felt they needed from us in order to continue to grow. We talked about the future, and how different it would be if I were in the picture versus out of the picture. When you have a terminal diagnosis, it becomes easier to talk about things with eternal significance. Like what your family will be like when you are dead and gone. Most people shy away from these conversations, as if avoiding them can add days, weeks or years to their lives. Avoidance doesn't do that. It just keeps you from talking about the inevitable. A terminal diagnosis removes the last barrier and you communicate with your loved ones on a much deeper and more meaningful level.

The last meeting was with the pulmonologist. The spot in my lung that required a special bronchoscopy was still problematic. We still didn't know what it was. There were a lot of things it could be that weren't a problem. But there one thing that could be a huge concern. If it were a fungal infection then it could be potentially fatal during the prep for the stem cell transplant. During the week immediately preceding the transplant, you are given a regime called BEAM. This consists of four drugs called BCNU (also called Carmustine, Etoposide, Ara-c (Cytarabine) and Melphalan. These drugs completely wipe out your entire immune system, including any and all vaccinations you ever had, all the way back to childhood. Your body literally has *no* ability to fight infection of any kind.

A fungal infection is bad, really bad. Massey wanted to do their own CT of the spot, and possibly preventively treat it beforehand. The problem was, the drug to treat it, Voriconazole, was ridiculously expensive, and requests for it were routinely denied by insurance companies unless it could be definitively proven it was necessary. They would not pay for it "just in case." The team at Massey (and later at MD Anderson) are veterans of the insurance wars, and knew how to win, but it took time, and it was denied the first two attempts.

While we were fighting the insurance company, I continued the preparation. The staff ensures you are medically able to withstand the procedure. Months earlier I had started walking every day, and had gotten up to five miles a day, every day, without fail. Do you know how oranges become oranges? By hanging in there! I hung in there and walked every day, whether it was raining, snowing, wind blowing or hailing. No matter what, I was out there every day.

Massey did their own CT scan on December 21. Literally an hour and half there and an hour and a half back for a 4-minute procedure. When I got home, I was able to continue what has become a holiday tradition for my family. We make chocolate pinwheel cookies, and only at Christmastime. My kids fight over the cookies, and over the pieces of the dough/roll that comes apart. I make about 35 dozen and they are usually gone in a few days. A few years back I started hiding some in the freezer for me to have, but they discovered that secret as well. It is a long and involved two-day process, but it's a labor of love. I never enjoyed making them as much as I did then.

Every year at Christmastime I would invite every single person on staff at Saint Luke, and their spouses or significant others over for dinner. That Christmas I decided I was going to do it again, even though my immune system was compromised. I wore a mask the whole evening, and stayed away from handshakes and hugs, and we had a roaring time during our Dirty Santa exchange.

We got great news on December 23. My insurance company

had finally relented and agreed to pay for the Voriconazole. The medical staff was primarily concerned that the spot that wouldn't go out was a fungus called aspergillosis. Aspergillosis is caused by a common mold that lives indoors and outdoors. Most people breathe it in every day and have no problem. But it is particularly nasty for those with compromised immune systems. In addition to the Voriconazole I was also put on a special antibiotic. Antibiotics attack bad bacteria, but they also destroy good, which can be even more worrisome when you are immunocompromised. Both of these medications come with serious side effects and I was going to have to have additional blood, liver, kidney and heart function tests run while taking them.

I was also warned that during the "loading phase" (when you first start taking a new medicine), many people experienced serious vision issues, and I was advised to be on guard for that.

Little did I know what I was in for! I have read reports of people who had a drug trip while taking LSD or some other hallucinogenic. I now have first-hand experience just how vivid that can be. I had been on the Voriconazole for a full day, and that night, while sleeping, I started tripping. I woke up and jumped out of bed, almost breaking my cello. Our bookcase and window in our bedroom appeared to me to be life size nutcrackers that were coming after Clara, and I jumped up to protect her. The clarity with which I saw these was amazing. It was as though I had 20/10 vision or better. They then melted into the room, and on the wall a series of letters and numbers appeared. It seemed to be a code of some sort, but one I could just not quite make out. The ceiling turned into a giant 3D relief map of the world, that looked like it had been drawn by da Vinci. All of these images were as real as real could be, and were crystal clear to me, and I can remember them in minute detail now six years later.

I finally went back to sleep and had the most vivid dreams of my life. One summer Clara and Taylor went on our church's mission trip to Brazil. In the lead-up to that they had to take medicine to prevent Malaria. Both of them said it gave them the most vivid dreams they had ever had. I now understood what they meant. I had the most colorful, vivid dreams I've ever had.

The next morning was Christmas Eve. Taylor had come home from college and needed to run out and do some last-minute shopping so I offered to go with him. Before we left, I stopped in our downstairs bathroom. When I turned on the light and closed the door the grout between the floor tiles turned a bright sparkling purple. It was literally sparking like a sparkler you would light and wave on the fourth of July. I opened and closed the door several times, and each time I closed the door, there was the bright sparkly purple. When I opened the door, it was its normal dingy grout color. I told Taylor that for both of our sakes it would be better if he drove.

Later that evening I was driving to our 7:00 p.m. Christmas Eve service. Next to Easter, this is always our highest attended service of the year, and I was thrilled I had to chance to lead it once again. On the way there I started hallucinating again, and the branches of the trees over the road appeared to me to be huge intersecting and interconnecting train tracks. I was scared, it was all so real. I was thankful the church was only a mile from home, and I managed to get there without any incident, although I took my own driving privileges away. I didn't want to endanger myself or anyone else.

When I got to church, I parked in my normal pastors spot near the door and walked in. I've never been a fan of florescent lights, detesting them to the point I think their inventor has their own rung in hell. I don't like the way they make me feel, I never have. That night was even worse, because the lighting caused everyone's hair to appear to be a vivid purple. Depending on people's actual hair color, there were various shades, but everyone had purple hair. I stood on the stage of The Grove, which was the main part of the huge addition we had recently completed, preparing to lead almost 500 people at once, and every one of them had purple hair. I also could not feel my feet, and was very unsteady. At the time I was wearing a special shoe called Vibram five finger (five toed shoe), and were it not for that I am sure I would have lost my balance. The thought quickly went through my head—"When you stumble, make it part of the dance." I was determined to dance. When it came time for the communion liturgy, I could not remember if I had recited the part about the Cup, right when we got to the end of it. My mind raced a million miles an hour and the thought came to me that if in fact I had forgotten to recite that part, probably only a handful of people would know. But if I recited it twice in a row *everyone* would know. I decided to chance it that I had, in fact recited it (I found out later I had), but at the time it seemed like the most momentous decision. The last hymn sung every Christmas Eve is "Silent Night." Everyone lights a candle; the lights are turned off and it is the most holy beautiful moment of the year. When we turned off the lights and everyone held up their candle, I just started crying uncontrollably. I didn't care. I was overcome with emotion for being able to be there and to experience this Holy moment one more time. The candles all looked more like sparklers than candles. I had my son drive me home after service, because I was still hallucinating. But I was home safe, with all the people I loved around me, and all was right with my world.

The next day was Christmas. My children have always been wonderful on Christmas morning. One person opens a gift, and then they pick one out for someone else, then that person does the same. We often stop part way through to have breakfast, and then resume after we've eaten. We went through our normal ritual and when we were all done Brandon stood in the middle of the family and said, "I have a question. You are all here, and it's one of you, so I want whomever it is to tell me they did it." He then proceeded to tell us how, when he was in elementary school, he would often not eat his Little Debbie snack cake that Clara would put in his lunch, but would bring it home and put it in a Tupperware like container. He then hid it in a special hiding place he had found in the room he shared with Taylor. One day he discovered it was missing, and he never said a word about it because whomever took it never said a word about it either. We were all laughing so hard. The more he talked about it the more animated he got and the more we all laughed! It was the best Christmas ever. No one ever did admit being the guilty party, although the next year Clara gave Brandon and only Brandon a box of Little Debbie treats.

Christmas night I wrote on Caring Bridge: "While I would not wish this Inglorious Bastard on anyone, it has brought more blessings than curses. It has given me pause to consider what is truly important in life and what is not. It has made me cherish each day and every moment far more than before. It has brought my family closer together. Clara and I have deepened our relationship, vows and bond and have had many in-depth and long conversations about life, death, and love. It has brought me closer to God. It has forced me to consider my mortality, it has restructured my priorities. It has reconnected me to long lost friends and brought a host of new ones. It has dropped me to my knees in tears (often) but allowed me to see joy more often. It has given me time to right some wrongs. I have learned yet again the virtue of forgiveness. I'm more comfortable with eternity."

I closed that entry by saying a heartfelt "Thank you" to the IB, and gave it permission to leave now.

Of course, it wouldn't leave on its own, and we began actively getting ready for the stem cell transplant.

On January 5th I was taken off the Voriconazole because of elevated liver enzymes. I was switched to a new anti-fungal medicine that I was to receive intravenously at home every day. Being the caregiver is harder than being the patient in many ways, and this last item was certainly that for Clara as she cannot stand the sight of needles. Now, she was going to have to be the one to administer the new drug every day. Driving way out of her lane, she did just that, after being trained by a home health nurse. It was a time of high anxiety for me and everyone in my family. My life depended on getting the transplant, and the transplant hinged on getting rid of what we thought was a fungal infection. The decision was made medically that if it had not grown we would proceed with the transplant. I agreed to this—actually I suggested it. The medical team agreed! We would undergo the transplant first since I was ready for it, and we would deal with the spot later. It was being carefully watched and monitored though.

I had passed all the organ testing, only one last thing was required. I had to pass a cardiac stress test. This is where they put you on a treadmill, gradually increase the speed and angle, and monitor your heart rate. I had to be able to get my heart rate to eighty percent of its maximum, and keep it there for twenty minutes.

The day came for the test and we once again went to Massey. Self-driving cars were making news around this time, and I remarked to Clara that our van could probably go to Massey and back without a driver just from muscle memory.

I got on the treadmill and started walking. At last we got to my target heart rate, and I had to keep going for twenty minutes. I just went away to a happy place in my head and didn't even notice the passing of time, except when the assistant would call out "five minutes," "ten minutes," etc. I wasn't about to get knocked out of the transplant for this, and what they didn't know was I could have gone an hour, or two hours or longer. I was thinking about going to my son and daughter's college and high school graduation, I was envisioning helping my daughter move into her college dorm. I thought good positive happy thoughts about the future memories I would be able to have, and honestly didn't even feel tired. When the twenty-minute mark came I let out a holler of joy that I am sure could have been heard throughout the hospital. I had finally met all the qualifications for the stem cell transplant, and we were going up to the bone marrow unit to sign consent forms. It was one of the happiest days I had since I had been diagnosed.

For three consecutive days we drove the ninety-minute journey to and from Massey just to receive an injection of a drug called Neupogen. Neupogen helps to reduce the risk of infection in cancer patients who are receiving strong chemotherapy that decreases the number of infection-fighting white blood cells.

Stem cells are brilliant little creatures. They can become anything in your body. Depending on what you need, the same stem cell could become a brain cell, or a toenail. They literally are what makes us, us during our natal growth and development.

They are also very much "momma's boys" and "daddy's girls." That is, they don't want to leave home (the bone marrow) unless they are kicked out of the nest. And even then, they try their hardest to rebound and come back. I remarked to the docs that the stem cells sounded very much like adult children. They can become whatever they want, but they like to stay at home, or come back home. They told me I nailed it with that analogy!

My case manager called me to say my cell counts were not high enough and I had to go and get a shot of Mozobil. This was the newly approved drug my nephew Jason had told me about that allowed me to be my own donor, which eliminated all the risks and side effects of rejection from a different donor.

The Mozobil moves the stem cells out of the marrow and into the blood stream so they can be collected for an "autologous" transplant. Autologous simply means you are your own donor.

The first thing I had done after diagnosis was to have a mediport installed in my chest. This allows for the administering of chemotherapy, blood draws, etc. without having to have a needle stick each time. Many of the drugs used are also so powerful that the small vessels in your arm often can't handle them. The mediport is accessed by a needle into it to administer whatever you are receiving, and it empties into the body through one of the large veins in the heart.

I traveled to Richmond and had a second catheter installed in my chest to collect the stem cells. A sense of humor is a must when dealing with cancer, so I referred to these two things hanging from my chest, as my "chesticles."

The collecting of the stem cells is a painless and miraculous process. It is like giving blood or receiving a transfusion. Actually, it's both of these. For an autologous stem cell transplant, the cells are obtained from the patient's own blood. For an allogenic transplant, the stem cells are obtained from a tissue-matched donor who may be related or unrelated. Blood is collected via a catheter and passed through a special machine that separates the stem cells from the rest of the blood. The remaining blood is then re-injected into the donor. The transplant team makes the decision for each patient how many cells need to be collected. For me it was five million. I have no idea how the number of stem cells are counted, but after the first day we had not collected enough so I had to return for a second day. The morning of the third day my case manager called and said collection was successful, and we had over seven and a half million cells. These were frozen and would be reinjected into me after I underwent the strong chemo regime that wipes out your immune system and your bone marrow.

I went home and got busy. I ground thirty-eight pounds of pork butt and made my grandfather's kielbasa recipe. Then I ground eighteen pounds of venison and made venison sausage. My family really loves them both, and I didn't know if I would ever get another chance to make them, so I made as much as our freezer could hold. I also gave a lot away to friends, doctors, nurses, anyone that wanted some.

I got our tax information to our accountant months earlier than usual, and made beef brisket, something my family loves. It takes twenty-six hours to make, but it is so worth it!

It was a time of high stress and anxiety, so doing normal things like making sausage and preparing taxes was my way of coping. I also realized that we had close to thirty accounts that had passwords, and they were all in my head and Clara didn't know them. I made a list of every account, our username and password and put it in our safe. I hoped she would not need it for many years, but I also wanted to make things as easy on her as I could.

All that was needed now was for a bed to open up on the bone marrow transplant unit. On January 23rd a bed became available and I was admitted. Clara and I drove to Richmond the night before and stayed at a fancy hotel. We went out to dinner at the most expensive steak house in Richmond and ordered a bottle of wine that cost more than I ever paid for a single bottle before or since. The next morning when I got out of the shower I shaved my head. I knew the chemo was going to make me bald, and so rather than let it, I did it myself. When your life is spinning out of control, taking charge of the little things you can control helps to lessen the stress and uncertainty.

I went through a six-day process of intense chemotherapy that totally destroyed my immune system. On the seventh day I rested (how biblical) and the eighth day I received my stem cells back in a procedure that took about an hour. January 31, 2017.

This "re-birthday" is also known as Day 0. Everything that would come after depended on how many days I was out post-transplant.

I was walking 10,000 steps a day, or five miles. The bone marrow unit consisted of three long hallways, with the nurses' station in the middle. I discovered that seven laps around all three wings equaled a mile, and so I walked thirty-five laps every day, pushing my infusion pole, which Clara named "Harvey" along with me. Whenever I saw someone else walking, I would stop and encourage them. The staff started calling me "the hall walker." But that was the best thing I could do for myself to speed my recovery.

I was getting chemo four times a day and walking five miles, and these things took up most of the waking hours of each day. I had to put on a mask, gown and gloves every time I left my room, and every time someone came in, they had to dress that way also. Only my immediate family and the medical staff was allowed in as I was in isolation. There were two murals on the second hallway that I would stop and read every lap. The first said, "I didn't say it would be easy, I said it would be worth it." The second said, "Don't stop when you are tired, stop when you are done." I took both of these to heart thirty-five times a day.

The third night of chemo was eventful. One of the bags got a hole in it so we couldn't use it. We only had a one-hour window to get another one to keep on what was a tightly scripted and controlled schedule. The pharmacy wasn't able to get it to us in time, so we had to completely redo my schedule.

I set a few short-term goals. The first was to get out of the hospital. The second was to go home. The third was to get back to work, and the fourth was to be able to make it to Laura and Taylor's graduations in May and June. There were about thirty other items on that first bucket list.

When I first heard of a bone marrow transplant many years

ago, I wondered how in the world they did it. Do they cut open your bones and scrape the marrow out and put new marrow in? Don't all of your bones have marrow, so do they have to do it to your entire body?

My machinations and imaginings about the process were completely off. My stem cells were replanted in my body through the catheter in my chest. These were in bags like you would get fluid in through an IV. A doctor had to puncture each bag, after multiple medical personnel confirmed my name and birthday and medical record number, and after the same folks carefully looked at each bag of stem cells and confirmed they were mine.

All my previously collected stem cells were reintroduced into my body, and now we had to hope they would re-graft themselves and begin making new marrow.

The first night I spent in the bone marrow unit I kept being awakened by Braham's Lullaby playing periodically. There seemed to be no specific time this would happen, and it really irritated me.

The next morning I found out that every time a baby is born in the hospital, Braham's Lullaby is played on every floor. My outlook and attitude changed completely. What a beautiful gesture! I suggested to the staff that they also play it whenever someone goes through a bone marrow transplant, as we were in essence being re-born.

The last day of chemo arrived. I was given a very high dose intense drip of Melphalan. It is highly toxic and eliminated through the skin. I had to wear special protective clothing and had to shower often.

Day 0 was upon me—My re-birthday! For the rest of my life, everything will date from January 31, 2017.

Clara and Laura surprised me by printing a ton of photos of all our family over the years. They put these in cute frames and hung them on every available inch of my walls. It was a very visible reminder that I was surrounded by my family throughout this whole process.

After the transplant I was in a tremendous amount of pain, but I refused to stay in my bed. Every morning I would get up by 8:00, open my window shades and sit in the chair in my room. I did a lot of reading during those days. I was still walking five miles a day, even when I didn't feel up to it. One of the things I read during those first few days was this:

The universe
Is not trying
To break you
My dear,
It's trying
To find a way
To wake you up,
So that you
Will see
What is real,
And worth fighting for.
It takes time
To heal,
But it also
Takes courage

And courage was what I needed. I developed a severe case of mucositis. This is an inflammation and ulceration of the mucous membranes lining the digestive tract. For me, I also had it in my mouth and throat. It was very painful. I was told that most patients who receive high dose chemotherapy and a stem cell transplant are affected by this. My already limited diet got limited even more. I remember the dietitian coming in and giving me my choices for my meal—I could have oatmeal, grits, or cream of wheat. "What's the difference?" I exclaimed, "Just rotate between the three." The pain from the transplant and from the mucositis finally got to me and I agreed to go on a morphine pump. This helped greatly with staying on top of and managing the pain, but it made me listless and with no energy.

One day, Brandon and Laura came and surprised me. I think my beleaguered condition startled them, although neither one would say it. Chatting with them for twenty minutes completely wore me out, and it broke my heart to tell them I was too tired to continue the visit. They both jumped up and got out as fast as they could (or so it felt to me). I remember saying to myself, "No way, this is *not* how my kids are going to remember me." When you are called "dad," giving up is *not* an option! I put on a mask, gown and gloves and unplugged Harvey the med pole, and took him out in the hallway to walk. The staff was surprised to see me, but I told them what had just happened with my kids, and I was more determined than ever that I was going to beat this thing! I wasn't able to go five miles that day, but I did go one mile.

I had blood labs drawn every day, and usually I would need magnesium or calcium. But my numbers had gotten so low I needed a transfusion of platelets. As they were giving them to me, I developed a severe case of hives. That was an adventure! Between the Benadryl, hydrocortisone, steroids and morphine I got the best night sleep I had since I had been in the unit. I was woken up every four hours to get vital signs, and I don't even remember being awoken that night. That day/night was a *huge* turning point for me because of Laura and Brandon. I knew I had the inner strength and will to continue to fight hard, and I was supremely confident that not only was I going to fight, I was going to win!

6

"You Can't Wait Until Life Isn't Hard to be Happy."
~ Nightbirdie, Jane Marczewski

You do not need to know precisely what is happening, or exactly where it is all going. What you need is to recognize the possibilities and challenges offered by the present moment, and to embrace them with courage, faith and hope.
~Thomas Merton

As already stated my bone marrow transplant was on January 31, 2017 and called "Day 0." Everything that happens after that is dated from Day 0. I'm an extremely competitive person. My life long buddies and I compete in *everything*! So when I heard that the earliest anyone had been discharged from the residential unit was Day 14, I had a goal. And I let my doctors know I had that goal. A strong person is not the one who doesn't cry. A strong person is one who is quiet and sheds tears for a moment, and then picks up the sword and fights again. I was ready to continue on to the next stage of recovery, which was discharge from the hospital.

Once I was able to be discharged from the hospital, I was going to have to stay within five minutes of the bone marrow unit for thirty to sixty days. Given my transplant, if something went wrong, I couldn't just go to an emergency room, I had to get to the bone marrow clinic.

A dear friend, George Emerson, owned an apartment

building about six blocks from the main hospital, and graciously gifted Clara and me the use of one of the apartments for as long as we needed it. He told me he would trade the rent with me for prayers for him and his partners. What a wonderful gift he gave us, as housing costs were not covered by insurance and would surely be many thousands of dollars.

I was discharged on Day 13. I had set a new record and I was proud of myself. I knew I had to set small goals all along the way if I was to reach my ultimate goal. In addition to being no more than thirty minutes from the Bone Marrow unit, I also had to have a caregiver stay with me 24/7. Being babysat is not easy for me, but at least my primary caregiver was Clara. The risk of infection was so high that I was not allowed to cook or clean up (the latter being just fine actually). I was not even allowed to pick up something that had fallen on the floor. Someone else had to do it, and then it needed to be disinfected. I couldn't wear any clothes, underwear or socks for more than a day and my sheets and towels had to be washed daily. That was a lot of extra work asked of my caregiver, and as always Clara did it lovingly and willingly, although I could see the strain of stress and uncertainty in her. She has always been a "do-er" and while these additional tasks gave her that outlet, I am sure she would have just as welcomed a nap, or a book, or a day at the spa. But instead of any of these, she chose to take care of me.

Eating was difficult. Like a toddler, I had to have each new food introduced to me slowly, one at a time to see if I could tolerate it. Everything was bland and had to be cooked to well done. I tried to imagine each bite of oatmeal as being a thick juicy steak, but I failed at fooling myself. It was definitely oatmeal.

Clara kept reminding me, this is temporary, you can get through this. The more I exercised and drank fluids, the faster I would recover. Three times a day I would put on a face mask and gloves and walk every floor and every staircase of the apartment building. I think I creeped out some of the permanent residents as they wondered who was this constant ghost-like hall walker? But I got to know the building and the residents well. I didn't know their names or faces, but I know who ordered Amazon Prime all the time, who got food delivered frequently. I even knew who smoked marijuana and when.

My new "new normal" routine was established. Every day I would go to the clinic in the morning for an extensive blood draw. Then I would go sit in a big leather chair in the infusion room and wait for the results. Then they would give me "replenishments." Usually I needed magnesium and potassium every day. Twice I needed platelets, but that was early on.

Then I would go back to the apartment and force myself to eat and exercise. I was up to six miles a day—two miles, three times a day.

The wonderful thing about being in the apartment was that our son Taylor arranged his schedule at the University of Virginia so that he could be with me on weekends. This allowed Clara to go back home and lead worship, take care of whatever needed to be done at the house or with the kids and have some time to herself that wasn't about taking care of me. The back and forth was taking a toll on both of them, but I knew they were doing it out of love. The fact my son would give up weekends at college during his final semester spoke volumes to me about his maturity level and the man he had become, and was I ever proud.

The head of the bone marrow transplant unit, Dr. John McCarthy, told me that a transplant like mine ages a person twenty years. Diet, exercise and hydration are all keys to reducing this number. I was working hard at all of them, and was laser focused on completely beating this Inglorious Bastard. So I basically entered the hospital aged 59 and came out 79. But it was a good looking 79, if I do say so myself!

After two weeks of daily trips to the clinic, Dr. McCarthy gave us the good news that I could scale back my visits to Mondays and Thursdays. This was another big milestone on the way to my goal of coming home. Dr. McCarthy gave me a date for that—March 13, 2017. Day 41. I had been told the record for being able to go home was forty days, and I would have beat that except for the weekend. I would take it!

The weekend of March 4 was especially beautiful. In addition to having Taylor, my third son Brandon came to see me and spend the night. Brandon was so exhausted when he showed up that he just went into my bedroom and fell asleep for hours, but that was okay with me. I just cherished having him close by. The lymphoma had taught me a lot of lessons, one being that short moments can make long memories. Rachel Marie Martin wrote —"Sometimes you have to let go of the picture of what you thought life would be like and learn to find joy in the story you're living." I was doing just that.

On March 6th we met with another of the lead doctors, Dr. Harold Chung. He looked over my chart and the progress I had made since being discharged and said, "Why are you still here? You can go home." Clara and I just sat there stunned, not sure we had heard him correctly. I remember her saying, "Home, like today home?" Dr. Chung simply replied, "Yes, today." I had done it! I had set a new record. The old record of going home after forty days was replaced with my new one of thirty-four days.

The next few hours Clara frantically packed, cleaned the apartment and got everything ready for us to go home. I had made the trip from Massey to Yorktown so many times that it became rote. But this trip was anything but rote, I was going home *for good*.

When we got home, before we even went inside, Clara

and I took a selfie of the two of us. It was probably the most joyous picture we've ever taken together, even if my head was totally bald. Throughout the process in addition to losing my hair, I also lost fifty-seven pounds. I always told people I don't recommend the diet I went on to lose so much weight.

Finally coming home was such a blessing. To sleep in my own bed every night felt like such a gift. But it was also a challenge, because while I was in familiar surroundings, *everything* was different. I was still under so many precautions and limitations. I couldn't cook anything. I couldn't clean up anything (although for this one I bet if you were to ask Clara or one of the kids if it were a restriction or a limitation, you'd no doubt be met with a quizzical look). I could not touch anything outside, and I had to wash my hands constantly. Public Service Announcement—frequent hand washing is the single most effective barrier to avoiding germs that anyone can do. Most of the bad bacteria and germs get on our body on our hands, and into our body when we rub our eyes, or nose or mouth. The simple act of hand washing and being aware of what your hands come into contact with can reduce your risk of illness or infection significantly.

Still my clothes and towels had to be washed every day, and I had to wear a mask and gloves anytime I went anywhere. I had to stay away from crowds, I couldn't go to stores or restaurants. March 19, 2017 was a memorable day as I was able to lead worship for the first time in over two months. I had to avoid contact with everyone and asked everyone to keep their distance. I wore a mask the whole time, but things were moving in the right direction. So many things about the healing process were out of my control, so I learned to just focus on those things that were in my control—namely diet, hydration and exercise. I kept telling myself, "Do whatever is next." I was supposed to drink a minimum of 128 ounces a day (think 15, 8 oz. glasses). The chemo that took away my immune system also dehydrates the body for many months and counter acting that was something within my power.

Next to hydration, exercise is the number one thing that helps the recovery process. My energy level fluctuated a lot from day to day, but I walked at least four miles a day, every day, rain or shine. I remember one day that was so windy I called Clara to come pick me up and she could barely hear what I was saying because of the wind. Thanks to the "share my location" feature of our phones she was able to find me.

After one of my daily walks, I came home and wrote in my journal:

> **"Life keeps leading us on journeys we would never go on if it were up to us. Don't be afraid. Have faith. Find the lessons. The path isn't a straight line; it's a spiral. You continually come back to things you thought you understood and see deeper truths."**

During the last days of March, we got the results from then latest CT scan. The spot on my right lung was still there and had grown, even despite the high dose chemotherapy I had gone through before transplant. The chemo totally eliminated my immune system, but this sucker was still there. I remember actually talking to this spot out loud during my walk. "You're tough and you're resilient you little bastard, I'll give you that." (Note, if you're bothered by the earthy language realize that the word "bastard" can mean a number of things, one of them being *"(of a thing) no longer in its pure or original form; debased."* It is this meaning I have in mind when I refer to cancer as the Inglorious Bastard, or IB). "You may be resilient, but I'm more resilient! You may be tough, but I'm tougher! I *am* going to discover your true identity, and then I am going to evict you!"

And I believed that. I tell people that no one ever beat cancer thinking they couldn't ("well, what do you know, I beat the cancer, I didn't think I could do it!", said no one ever). Rather, you have to believe, down to the molecular level of your being, that you are going to defeat it.

There is a fundamental difference between hoping and believing. You have to train your body, mind and soul to believe, down to the very molecules that make up your essence, that you will defeat the cancer, no matter the odds! It takes the exact same amount of time and energy to imagine wonderful things as it does to worry, and the results are incredibly different. Remember, if there is a one in a million chance of surviving it, *someone* has to be that one. Why not you? Believe it!

Remember the Universal Law of One.
We are all connected.
Meaning, as I heal myself and raise my vibration others collectively benefit from that energy.

We met with the team at Massey in early April. Whatever it was in my lung, it was growing, despite being hit with Voriconazole, Posaconazole, and all the immune system killing chemo I had been given prior to transplant. Since nothing else had worked, we had to go to the option of last resort, which was surgery. We made the decision to go ahead with a lobectomy. Your lungs are nowhere near identical, and are considered two separate organs in terms of cancer and cancer traveling. Your left lung has two lobes, your right lung three. The surgeon said that more than likely they would need to remove the entire upper lobe of my right lung to get it. I have always had huge lungs and whenever I get a chest x-ray the technician has to take two pictures to get them all, so I felt I would still have plenty of lung function even with a third of the right one removed. After meeting with the surgeon, we agreed to schedule it for April 17, which would give me plenty of time to recover enough to be able to attend Taylor's graduation from the University of Virginia on May 20. April 17 was also "Easter Monday." The first day after the resurrection. It seemed very fitting to me. My former Bishop, the beloved Charlene Kammerer, told me I didn't need to write an Easter sermon, that I could give powerful testimony to the resurrection just by showing up!

The surgery was supposed to take about three hours but ended up taking five and a half. Clara didn't exactly panic, mainly because Taylor surprised her and came to sit with her through it. The surgeon later gave her a measure of comfort when he told her the procedure took so long because he had a hard time finding the spot, it was so small. We still didn't know what the mass was, and wouldn't until the pathology report came back. Because of the recent bone marrow transplant I was isolated in a special room and kept away from other patients. I also had to start using what they called "breathing toys" six times a day. With one, you would take a normal breath and then blow out as long as you could and when you thought you couldn't go any farther, you were supposed to keep going. It was fascinating actually. Try it. Breathe in normally then breathe out through your mouth until you feel your lungs are empty then keep pushing. You will be surprised at the amount of air left in your lungs when you think you have emptied them. The other device was the opposite. You had to form a tight suction over it and inhale as deeply as you could against resistance. Like everything else in my recovery, I went after these with a vengeance. I told my doctor, "Don't tell me the minimum number of times a day I should do this, give me the maximum I shouldn't exceed." I was determined to regain my lung function so I could walk the lawn with my son when he wore the honor of honors at UVA.

Two days post-surgery and I went into Atrial Fibrillation

again (Afib). Afib is when the upper chambers of your heart beat rapidly with no discernible rhythm. It can be traumatic, or even deadly, because there is always the chance of throwing a clot. Blood clots (like scabs on your skin after a cut) form when your blood doesn't flow properly. If it pools in your blood vessels or heart, the platelets are more likely to stick together. Atrial fibrillation and deep vein thrombosis (DVT) are two conditions where slow moving blood can cause clotting problems. Because I had previous experience with both DVT and Afib, I was moved to cardiac intensive care. I had been in Afib for 13 hours with my heart beating 134 times a minute. I was as worn out as I've ever been.

Three days after surgery the surgeon came and removed the drainage tube that had been put in my chest. I remember him waking me up very early, so I wasn't sure if I was awake or dreaming. But once he started pulling that tube out, I knew from the pain I wasn't dreaming. I think I may have said a few words that shocked him, but man oh man did it hurt to have that pulled out! The day got much better when an old friend from seminary, Bubba Brock, came up from North Carolina to visit. Bubba had introduced me to Clara and was one of the pastors who presided at our marriage ceremony. It was great to catch up as it totally took my mind off the current pain.

I was moved to the step-down unit, room 444, which was interesting. A church member had sent me a card with an angel pin in it. The card read, "The recurring angel number 444 bears the meaning of honesty and inner-wisdom. Also, this is a sign that the angels are sending you encouragement. Therefore, you can continue to work hard and pursue your passions. Moreover, 444 represents your rigorous goal-seeking nature." Like a horoscope that seems to aptly fit, I chose to believe this. That night during dinner, I wrote on my place mat, "Eventually you'll stop calling them coincidences and realize how powerful you are."

I was at Day 80, looking forward to reaching Day 100 when a number of restrictions would be lifted.

On April 21, Taylor called to tell me he had been offered the job he really wanted. He already had another job offer in hand, and both before he graduated. As we were talking the nurse practitioner came in to tell me I was being discharged. What a joy for me to have these occur simultaneously, something I will never forget.

I was discharged and we anxiously waited for the report from the surgeon. I remember when my younger brother Dan was born my mother stayed 10 days in the hospital. I have 1/3 of my right lung removed on a Monday and I'm discharged on a Friday. Clara and I went for a walk when we got home, anxious about the results from the surgeon.

On April 28 the surgeon called with the pathology report. The spot on my lung turned out to be non-small cell squamous cancer with neuroendocrine differentiation. One of the deadliest lung cancers you can get, only occurring in 2-3% of lung cancer patients and almost exclusively in non-smokers. He said he was amazed we caught it when we did, that it is almost never caught at such an early stage, and both he and the tumor board felt the surgery was "curative," and that I would not need any chemo, radiation or further treatments as they got the margins they wanted by removing the lobe, and the cancer was not present at all in my lymph nodes. Had it not been for the lymphoma, we never would have discovered the lung cancer until it was probably too late. What I thought was my worst enemy (lymphoma), turned out to be my friend! Never be so sure of what you want that you wouldn't take something better. I suppose it would have been good if I never gotten lymphoma. But the lymphoma pointed me and my medical team to something far more deadly and sounded the alarm at the earliest possible time.

I thought I felt good enough to return to lead worship, at

least as the liturgist. But Clara put her foot down and emphatically said "No." I reminded her that I was still Senior Pastor of Saint Luke's and got the final say on things, especially worship. She reminded me she was the wife, which gave her the final word on *everything*. And she was not going to let me risk my health by engaging up close with upwards of 500 people in a morning! My argument that I'm the senior pastor and make final decisions fell apart to her argument that she was the wife who loved me and was looking out for the safety and health of her husband and the father of her children. Never be so sure of what you want (to lead worship) that you wouldn't take something better (the entire staff upping their game for worship to cover my absence.). To the surprise of no one with the possible exception of the "macho" men, Clara won that argument handily. Love always wins.

7

Most of the Shadows in Life Come From Standing in Your Own Sunshine
~Ralph Waldo Emerson

You're not going to master the rest of your life in one day. Just relax. Master the day. Then just keep doing that every day.
~Author Unknown

We/I had our sights set firmly on Day 100 which for me was May 11, 2017. Day 100 is the biggest day in the life of someone who has undergone a stem cell or bone marrow transplant, as that is the day you can begin to walk down the path of normal again. Although spoiler alert here. Your "old normal" and your "new normal" may be so different that they don't recognize each other.

Don't be afraid to start over again. This time you're not starting from scratch, you're starting from experience.

Of course, I was still actively healing from having the upper third of my right lung removed on April 17. But I was healing, and was bound and determined to use the story of my healing to help others facing a similar story.

"I love when people who have been through hell, walk out of the flames carrying buckets of water for those still consumed by the fire." ~Stephanie Sparkles

Day 100 arrived. I eagerly awaited this day much as a child anticipates the arrival of Santa Claus. May 11, 2017—I had finally gotten my get out of jail free card. I had been working exclusively from home since my return, to avoid the 50,000 square foot church that was active day and night, and which houses a morning preschool. I was now going to be allowed to return to my office in the afternoons, after preschool let out. I still had to take precautions like wearing a mask in public, being super conscious of touching hands or what my hands touched.

A little over a week past Day 100, Day 109 to be exact, I was able to be present for one of my top bucket list items. The thought of being at this day is what gave me the inner drive to get my walking up to four miles a day after my lung surgery. Day 109 for me was in essence Day 0 for Taylor as he was graduating from college and beginning a new phase of life. I watched him "walk the lawn" during final exercises at the University of Virginia, wearing "the honor of honors." I could not stop crying, nor did I even try. I was overcome with emotion. Pure, raw, from the bottom of my soul emotion poured out of me as my son walked past me in a black robe with cords draped around his neck and a mortar board on his head. Later in the day I got to sit in the University Chapel and watch him receive the diploma for which he had worked so hard. I thought again about how he gave up weekend partying his last semester of college so he could stay with me so Clara could go home to lead worship. If ever a father has been more proud of his son than I was of Taylor at that moment, I haven't made his acquaintance.

The Transfiguration of Jesus is a story told in three Gospels where Jesus is transfigured and becomes radiant in glory upon a mountain. Peter wants to capture and memorialize the moment by building three booths, one for Jesus, one for Moses and one for Elijah. But Jesus says no to the building project. As Jesus knew, and as generations of youth, and generations of adults would learn over the centuries, one simply cannot stay at a mountain top experience. Faith is renewed on the Mountaintop, but it's lived in the Valley.

When I was first diagnosed with Mantle Cell Lymphoma, I met with the Staff Parish Relations (SPRC) Committee at Saint Luke's. This is the committee that oversees all staff, both clergy and lay. This is also the committee that makes recommendations to the Bishop and Cabinet about the pastoral leadership needed by the church. I had several options. I could go on six-month medical leave, which would end my appointment with Saint Luke's, and a new Senior Pastor would be appointed. I could retire, although the early retirement penalties imposed on the required clergy pension annuity would be draconian. Or I could stay on as Senior Pastor during all the treatment. The SPRC committee was unanimous. They wanted me to stay on as senior pastor, and continue to collect my salary and have me and my family covered by our conference's excellent health insurance. I was grateful, extremely grateful, but not surprised. Saint Luke's was a church that knew how to love a senior clergy person and their family through a devastating illness. As previously mentioned, in 2011, on his 49th birthday the Director of Discipleship for Saint Luke's, Rev. James Pace, was diagnosed with leukemia. I requested the SPRC keep James on full time and allow him to continue to receive his full salary and benefits. They whole heartedly agreed. James died on Sunday (fitting, if you knew James) July 1, 2012, just six days shy of his 50th birthday. I knew James well enough to know how important it was to him that he be an active clergy member as he died. I also knew the denominational benefits plan well enough to know they would provide a nice college scholarship for his daughter when that time came, if he was still in the active relationship. Even though James was rarely in the building during that year, I never once heard a single complaint or question about what we were paying him, or why we were paying him. The Church loved him and his family through their darkest days in all the ways they could. Not only did they keep me on full time, they also gave me a hefty raise, knowing my family would be facing mounting medical bills. My family felt like we were in a dark valley, but my church pulled us out, if not to the mountaintop, then at least out of the valley where the spring waters were raging.

The one-year anniversary of my diagnosis came and was a time of deep reflection as well as deeper gratitude. In just a year's time I had been diagnosed with Stage IVb mantle cell lymphoma and had gone through six rounds of targeted chemotherapy. After three rounds I miraculously reached NED (No Evidence of Disease) which qualified me for a bone marrow transplant. I endured the transplant and was "re-birthed" on January 31, 2017. In April I had one third of my right lung removed. A year later I was in total remission from the lymphoma and the lung surgery was deemed curative. I was in the best shape of my adult life, physically, mentally, emotionally and spiritually. I posted to my Caring Bridge site that I intended the post on my one-year anniversary to be my last post for a long, long time. And it was, depending on how you define "long."

It wasn't long before my "new normal" resembled my "old normal" almost entirely. Someone once said,

"If you continue to carry the bricks from your past, you will end up building the same house that fell before."

I was back at work full time, which in a church can means north of 60-70 hours every week, most nights and every weekend. I had lost fifty-seven pounds and my once straight hair was now ridiculously curly, but other than those outward signs, there was very little difference in my daily life and stress pre-cancer and post treatment. I struggled with energy and would often work at home. But for the church and for my staff that was nothing new as I usually did sermon researching and writing out of the office. It borders on the impossible to compose and write a sermon in a church as active as Saint Luke's because of the constant interruptions. Often, the interruptions *are* the ministry, but often they are just breaking up any continuity of thought.

My energy level fluctuated greatly. Some days I could go full bore all day like I used to every day. Other days it was an effort to get dressed and leave the house. The greatest act of faith those days was to simply get up and face another day. I was in a three-year, post-transplant clinical trial to ascertain if an every-other month low dose of Rituximab was the best protocol to keep the lymphoma in the NED state. One thing was certain, it kept all my red and white counts at low levels, sometimes dangerously low. It also meant I could not be re-immunized with my childhood immunizations that had been wiped out by the pre-transplant chemo regimen. There were times when my energy level was so low I had to just close my office door, sit back in one chair with my feet up on another, and take a hard nap. These never lasted long as my phone would buzz from the Administrative Assistant, another staff member, or someone would knock on my door.

Throughout my career I had an open-door policy, and my staff knew what my door meant. If it was wide open, anyone could come in for any reason and I would stop what I was doing to talk about whatever they wanted to talk about. If my door was part-way open, it meant it was OK to come in if it was something of significance, but it also meant I was already working on something significant. I often said to my staff and others, "Whatever you bring to me is obviously important, or you wouldn't be bringing it to me. And while it is the most important thing to you, it might not be the most important (or highest priority) to me." Surprisingly, that is a hard concept for some people to understand. I have lost count of the hundreds of times people have walked into my office and started talking without even taking a moment to inquire, "Is this a good time?" There are a lot of skills one needs to be an effective senior pastor, and flexibility, compartmentalization, and prioritization are three.

I vividly remember one morning when a woman from the community had come to me, in tears and scared. She was afraid that her estranged husband was going around town with a power-of-attorney she had signed years earlier, and was taking her name off of all their financial accounts. I called a lawyer who was a member of the church and he advised me to bring her over right away, that moment, with no delay. As we were walking out of my office a church member stopped me by the arm to tell me there was a preschool mom in the parking lot who had a flat tire, and this church member was certain that if I, as senior pastor, went out and changed the woman's tire for her, that she would become a member of the church. I could tell the church member was angry with me and really didn't understand why rushing out of the door with this other person was a higher priority to me than stopping to change the tire. The church member got very indignant when I suggested that perhaps *they* change the tire for the woman. They even said out loud for all to hear, "What do you think this woman thinks of a church where the senior pastor won't come out and help her in her moment of need." Responding and not reacting is another vital skill for a senior pastor so I kept going with the woman I was taking to the lawyer.

After four months away I thought I knew what I was getting back in to. But in those four months, not only had my world changed drastically, so did our country. The polarization and partisanship that was seen on the nightly news was very evident daily, both in our community and in the church. The Bible has some specific things to say about the treatment of foreigners in your land, how we are to treat those we perceive as being "other," and about equality as human beings, among other controversial topics. When I would preach on any of those topics, a certain segment of Saint Luke's accused me of "putting politics ahead of the Gospel". Like in most churches, the people complaining didn't talk *to* me, they talked *about* me. When I preached a sermon on Matthew 18:15-17 which deals with how to handle conflict in the Church (i.e., if your brother or sister sins against you, go and talk to them in person, then bring one or two others...), people threatened to leave the church if I didn't stop being "political."

After a series of these threats, I invited several of the core members to join me in my office for coffee one Saturday morning. (I think they were shocked I knew who they were quite frankly). I had printed copies of a month of sermons and gave them each a copy. I asked them to read them, and to use a highlighter to highlight any sentence they felt was non-biblical, or was just political. After quickly looking through two of them one member of this group said to me, "You completely altered these. This isn't what you preached." I responded by saying that I never preach word for word from the manuscript, there are times when I ad-lib, but also knowing the vitriol that was in the church, the hateful things being said about me, I had been very intentional about staying close to script. Since our worship services are recorded, I offered to play them for them. The same person then said that I probably altered those as well! Thankfully, one of the other attendees, who was just as vocal most times reminded this person and others that the worship services were *video* taped, not just audio taped, and it would be pretty hard to alter them. I had the most vocal of the group pick which week to watch and we did. When it was over, I asked, "Please tell me what I said that wasn't Biblically grounded, or was just preaching politics." The most vocal one in the group stood up, threw his copies down on my conference table and said, "You might think this is what you said, you might even have some supposed video proof, but I guarantee you that's not what I heard on Sunday, and it's not what a lot of other folks heard on Sunday, and if you don't get back to the Bible, this place is going to get mighty empty!", and he stormed out.

There is an old adage I've repeated many times, "You can't put something in someone's head with reason when reason didn't take it out in the first place." Viktor Frankl, a survivor of Auschwitz wrote,

"Between stimulus and response there is a space... In that space is our power to choose our response. In our response, lies our growth and our freedom."

No response *is* a response. Sometimes it is also the best response.

Anxiety manifests itself a lot of different ways, as does grief. Well known to psychologists, anger is one of the primary ways that grief is expressed. Even though I knew that in my head, I was not at all prepared for the anger directed at me after my transplant and lung surgery.

Of course, everyone grieves differently. We all know that, at least intellectually, in our heads we know that. But in reality, somewhere in our psyche we have this belief that the way I am feeling about/understanding/processing an event or moment is the way everyone else around me is too. For the most part it is normal, and we don't even realize we are doing it.

Prior to my transplant and surgery, I would meet once a week for an hour with each of the full-time staff people. I had learned years earlier in my career that a church could grow only to the limit of the pastor's time, talent and energy. I also learned that those could be multiplied by hiring gifted and dedicated staff, and then staying out of their way. Our weekly meetings were a way to keep me up to date with ministries going on in the church, in the community and with our staff, without me having to micromanage everything. I always encouraged my staff to have "hard conversations." Quoting a colleague of mine I would often remind them, "We don't have hard conversations for the sake of having hard conversations. We have hard conversations to get to a better place." After serving at Saint Luke's for over eleven years, the staff knew I really meant this, and they were not afraid to have hard conversations with me, even if the hard part was talking to me or with me about something I disagreed with, or even, about me. I told my staff all the time that if they ever heard anything about themselves or their job for the first time in their annual review, then I wasn't doing my job. Any "course correction" direction should be given in real time, and not wait for an annual sit-down evaluation. I tried to model to them that this should be a two-way street, and that I was open to constructive criticism.

Whenever you are in a leadership position you will be criticized. When a candidate in a national election gets 55% of the vote, the pundits call it a "landslide!" After your first year serving a church, you are not going to get 100% approval rating. Unfortunately, many pastors take the parable of the lost sheep (Luke 15) and apply it to disgruntled parishioners, chasing after the one and leaving the ninety-nine. Far too much time is spent trying to sooth or appease someone who is not happy, rather than moving forward with ministry. I've often joked (but not joked at the same time) that, "Everyone in the church knows

I can't please everybody. And they are okay with that, as long as I please them!" If 55% is a landslide, then truly the best a pastor could hope for is a 60% "approval" rating (this is not the place for a long discussion on where a pastor's approval should come from. That topic alone could fill the pages of an entire book.) With that in mind it is indeed humbling to stand before a congregation to preach, knowing 40% of them probably wish it were someone else up there.

With the staff though, it's different. When a pastor has been at a church for a very long time, the staff begins to take on the characteristics of the pastor. The longer one is there, the more opportunity they have to hire new staff, or let them go. So over time the staff resembles the thinking, theology, and world view of the pastor, even more so, or at least sooner, than the rest of the church. Unlike an unhappy parishioner who will complain behind the pastors back, an unhappy staff member will either quit, resign, or be fired. Or make their unhappiness known in a hard conversation.

When I resumed my one-on-one weekly meetings is when I first got hit with the anger. I was not expecting it and it took me by surprise. One of my key staff members expressed in no uncertain terms how angry she was with me and how she fought with herself internally over this. She didn't think it was right to be angry with someone who discovered Stage IV cancer, yet at the same time, the uncertainty and anxiety it wrought, along with the countless daily questions all the staff had to answer about me in my absence did leave her feeling very angry with me. I realized this was not something I was going to be able to help her get over, and we both were going to have to learn anew how to work together in the midst of it. She also told me she was not the only staff member who felt that way.

Pastors are often confronted with the "anonymous army." When someone has a gripe and expresses it to the pastor, frequently they will attempt to bolster their argument by claiming "a lot of people" feel the same way. I learned early on in my career to be skeptical of comments like this. I had a hard and fast policy that both I and the church would not deal with any anonymous complaints. If someone slipped a note under my door the first thing I did was see if it was signed. If not, I threw it away without reading it. If someone had a complaint, they had to be mature enough and fair enough to attach their name to it. I had trained my staff and lay leadership that healthy churches deal with conflict in a healthy way, and the only healthy way to deal with conflict was face to face. A healthy church does not allow anonymous complaints to guide their decision making.

When I was told other staff people felt the same way, I was skeptical, but this also was not a person who bolstered her arguments with the anonymous army, so I had to take it seriously. That week at our full staff meeting I addressed the issue head on. I constantly preached to my staff, "Put it out when it is a match and it doesn't become a fire." Now it was time for me to heed my own advice. With the original staff persons permission, I shared with the full staff her feelings of anger towards me. I invited the rest of the staff to be honest and frank with me about their feelings during my extended absence and treatment, and gave them the option to either express their feelings out-loud in the full staff meeting, to share them with me one on one, or to write them down and give them to me. The only thing I asked was that they sign their name to it.

Several staff members took me up on the offer. Most of them had been on staff when James went through his year of dealing with leukemia, so having me diagnosed with lymphoma and all that meant had indeed put a tremendous strain and burden on them. Thankfully no one quit during this time, which was a real testament to them. I invited them all over to my house for dinner, and I purchased and grilled the highest-grade filet mignon I could find as a thank you for them keeping the ship on course during my absence. I also assured them it was OK to be angry.

In the coming weeks and months, I was able to work through all the issues my staff had with me and my situation, and didn't lose any of them, which is more a statement about who they are than who I am.

I shared with them this short poem by Mary Oliver:

Someone I loved
Once gave me
A box full of
Darkness.
It took me years
To understand
That this, too
Was a gift.

At the end of every year, all United Methodist pastors meet with their District Superintendent, or DS. For years I affectionately referred to this meeting as the, "Stay, Go, I don't care" meeting. Every United Methodist pastor is appointed every year. They are either reappointed to their current assignment, appointed to a new place, or could go either way. When I met with Seonyoung Kim, my DS, she suggested that I apply to go on medical leave. Clara and I had talked about this a lot, and the time was right. I didn't have the energy or stamina that serving a church required, and it was hard to attend to both my own healing while also running a church. We agreed that I would go on leave and Clara would seek a new appointment. She and I had worked together for sixteen years, and she had been an associate pastor her entire career. That was by choice as Clara often said, "The associate is THE minister" while the senior pastor is the "AD-minister." And truly, she was right.

When we first started in ministry, every year there would be an "announcement Sunday," when all the pastors in the conference would tell their churches if and where they were moving. Not only was this a terrible system because of the burden on the pastors and their children, it was usually also the worst kept secret in the church. It was better than the prior system where pastoral families would find out on the Sunday of annual conference if they were moving and then would have three days to pack their house, say goodbye to members and friends, move to a new church, and be in that pulpit the following Sunday. But it still didn't allow for a proper way to say goodbye, nor did it really allow the incoming pastor the time to say hello. We asked the DS for permission to tell the church right away. After serving Saint Luke's for twelve years, we had made a lot of friendships and connections, as had our children, and we wanted the time to properly say our goodbyes. This desire was granted and we let the church know I was going on medical leave and Clara was going to take a new appointment, but we didn't know where. It didn't take us long to find out.

Clara was called early on in the appointment making season, and asked to consider becoming the senior pastor of Chester United Methodist Church just south of Richmond. We had asked to be closer to Massey Cancer Center at Virginia Commonwealth University, and Clara had asked to not be appointed as an associate as she "didn't want to break in a new senior pastor." Chester UMC was the largest church in the James River District (1600+ members) with a very active community ministry, a large staff, and a full preschool. When we came to meet with the DS, he shared with us the "pastor profile" that Chester was looking for in their next pastor. Like the Bishop and Cabinet, when I read it over the very first person I thought of was Clara.

Thus, we entered a time of huge changes. I was no longer going to serve in an active role, and Clara was taking on a role she never sought. Despite being married for close to thirty years we had never picked out our own house. We always lived in church provided parsonages. Other than a bedroom suite we never even bought furniture, other than for the patio. During our fourth year at Saint Luke's we bought the parsonage and furnishings from the church, so now, in addition to packing for a move, we had to get our current house ready for sale, and buy one in Chester, while also saying our good-byes. Social scientists will tell you that changing jobs, relocating, and major medical issues are the highest stressors you can have—and we had them all. Thankfully we had a full-service Realtor in the church (Phil Jones) who not only handled the sale of our house, but also handled all the contracting work for the upgrades, repair and getting the house ready for sale. The first thing he told us was we had to get rid of at least half of everything in every room. We rented a storage facility and moved anything we thought we wanted to keep. The rest of our furniture we either gave away, sold, or took to the trash. When all of the remodeling was finished, we were down to half our master bedroom suite, two single mattresses on the floor of one of the other bedrooms, and two chairs and a table from the patio. We lived like that until we moved. For months we traveled to Chester traipsing through too many houses to count. Finally, with the help of a wonderful Realtor and member of Clara's new church (Julie Smart Koob), the offer we made on our dream home was accepted. The closings didn't match up with the start of Clara's ministry, so the chair of her Staff Parish Relations Committee let her stay with her and her husband while I stayed in Yorktown to finish the move and sale. We closed on our house in Yorktown one day, and two days later closed on the house in Chester. This was the first time we had ever chosen where to live. In all our previous moves Clara did most of the packing and unpacking. Now she was working full time and I wasn't, so it was yet another role reversal. When you move, boxes tend to multiply and no matter how many you unpack and put away, it seems you end the day with more than you started with. Taylor and his girlfriend Hannah came down the first couple of weekends to help us unpack, and their help was certainly welcome.

One afternoon three cars in a row drove by with the name of a local furniture company. We took that as a sign and went shopping. By the end of the night we had purchased every single piece of furniture for every room in the house, and also outdoors. We had been looking for a long time and knew what we wanted. Still, this in itself was quite a feat for us as we are such opposites we don't see the world the same way. I often say that we disagree about everything and Clara says we don't.

The summer of 2018 was spent moving in, unpacking, and getting to know the church and area. I had served my second appointment about 15 minutes from where we now lived. A number of church members from that church now were members at Chester, so we already knew a lot of people. Our new home had a pool and koi pond and those, as well as the acre+ yard kept me quite busy.

We went out to lunch after Clara's first Sunday and while there I got a phone call from a woman in Florida. She was the executor of my distant 2nd cousin Ruth's estate, and she called to tell me Ruth had left me a sizable portion of that estate. I had befriended Ruth over the last decade as we met on the Ancestry.com site. I would call her frequently and listen to all her stories about the Gestwick lore, and were there ever stories. Through the years she had sent me box after box of memorabilia from past generations of my family, knowing I would cherish it. I had helped her get a new phone when she dropped hers in the toilet late one night, and arranged for the "Geek Squad" to come to her house and repair her virus infected computer. I told Ruth that I wanted to die with no regrets and that the one regret I had was quitting piano lessons as a kid. Ruth stipulated she wanted me to buy a baby grand piano with some of the inheritance and get back to playing. Both of which I did. That piano is a thing of beauty and is my "go to" place of refuge from the storms. I can lose myself for hours and not once think about scans or needles or medicines or anything else that so competes for my head space.

One of the hardest things about moving occurred to us some time after we moved. While this new place was "home" for Clara and me, it never was and never will be for any of our children. Instead of it being "home," it is Mom and Dad's house. Our children were all in their late teens and early twenties, and we had lived twelve years in the same home in Yorktown, so their adaptation was even more stressful than mine and Clara's. Our youngest son Brandon took it the hardest, and throughout the first year in our new home, it was difficult and next to impossible for him to spend the night. He would get very emotional and leave. So many important changes had come at him and the other children all at once.

From the time we were dating and every year after, Clara and I and our children along with all her siblings, their spouses and their children would gather at her parent's home in Florence, South Carolina for Thanksgiving. The Friday after we would exchange Christmas presents with that side of the family. An older uncle named it "Thankxmas," and the name stuck. Remarkably, for over twenty-five years, every cousin, child and in-law made it every year, with very few exceptions. Instead of a turkey, we would have a "pig-pickin" and roast a whole hog for twenty-four hours or so. At first it was just the "grown-ups" (although I kind of balk at being in that category) who took turns watching the temperature, but as all the grandchildren (cousins) got older they took on more and more of the responsibility of sitting up all night tending to the roasting of the hog, and in the later years took over the late night and early morning rotations completely. As the cousins got older, moved up in school or off to college, it became harder and harder to get them all together. When our kids were young, we would load them all in to the minivan, and they would watch movies or play the alphabet game with highway signs. As they got older, we started coming in two, and then three and sometimes as many as four vehicles, but we all made it. Even through my diagnosis and treatment, even after my bone marrow transplant, I was able to make the family gathering. 2017 was the last time we all gathered for Thankxmas. Clara's father died in April of 2018, and her older brother took the house. The day Brandon got home from his epic road trip, literally, just a couple hours later I let all my children know I had been diagnosed with lymphoma, now his grandfather had died and the yearly tradition of all the cousins getting together had stopped. Like all of us, Brandon longed for "the good old days," and his grief over their loss came out in the way he perceived mine and Clara's new house.

"Life is not unlike cinema. Each scene has its own music, and the music is created for the scene, woven to it in ways we do not understand. No matter how much we may love the melody of a bygone day or imagine the song of a future one, we must dance with the music of today…"
~Lisa Wingate "*Before We Were Yours*"

Thankfully those difficult days are behind us. We still have not established a new holiday tradition with our now adult children, but I imagine as they graduate, marry and possibly have children of their own something new will be created.

8

There's No Education in the Second Kick of a Mule

Many want God's anointing...But they don't want the crushing that produces the oil.

Without rain, nothing grows. Learn to embrace the storms in your life. Just say the words, "September 11", or "9/11" and most people immediately remember the infamous day in American history when the Twin Towers in New York City came down. September 11, 2018 brought me into a new storm. The CT scan I had that day showed my lung cancer had come back in two places in my right lung. There was also a spot in my left lung that we weren't sure of. It could be an infection (I had a cough for months that wouldn't go away), or it could be cancer. While most people speak of their lungs as though they were one organ, actually they are vastly different from each other. When cancer moves between both lungs, it is no different than if it moved to a different organ. Now in addition to the cancer in my right lung, "something" was in my left. When physicians treat lung cancer, one of the first steps, and one of the most important things in treating cancer is the "staging."

Non-small cell lung cancer (NSCLC) staging uses the TNM system:
T (tumor): This describes the size of the original tumor.
N (node): This indicates whether cancer is present in the lymph nodes.

M (metastasis): This refers to whether cancer has spread to other parts of the body, usually the liver, bones or brain.

A number (0-4) or the letter X is assigned to each factor. A high number indicates increasing severity.

The stages of NSCLC are:

Occult-stage: Cancer cells are found in sputum, but no tumor can be found in the lung by imaging tests or bronchoscopy, or the tumor is too small to be checked.

Stage 0: Cancer at this stage is also known as carcinoma in situ. The cancer is tiny in size and has not spread into deeper lung tissues or outside the lungs.

Stage I (stage 1): Cancer may be present in the underlying lung tissues, but the lymph nodes remain unaffected.

Stage II (stage 2): The cancer may have spread to nearby lymph nodes or into the chest wall.

Stage III (stage 3): The cancer is continuing to spread from the lungs to the lymph nodes or to nearby structures and organs, such as the heart, trachea and esophagus.

Stage IV (stage 4): non-small cell lung cancer (NSCLC) is the most advanced form of the disease. In stage IV, the cancer has metastasized, or spread, beyond the lungs into other areas of the body. About 40 percent of NSCLC patients are diagnosed with lung cancer when they are in stage IV. The five-year survival rate for those diagnosed with stage IV lung cancer is less than 10 percent.

Because of all these factors, proper staging is absolutely key to deciding the course of treatment. Massey Cancer Center recommended I have the middle lobe of my right lung removed, and the lower lobe sectioned to remove the cancer. I wasn't keen on doing this, as there is a limited amount of lung tissue I can sacrifice before there is none left. Dr. Kessler, my lymphoma doctor agreed with me. He described NSCLC as being like grass seed. If you throw out a handful of seed, some will sprout up immediately, some a little later and some a lot later. The lung cancer we discovered in 2017 was the first to sprout. We also didn't know what it was until *after* the surgery. Even though he wasn't my lung doctor, Kessler was pretty insistent that I not go the surgery route, since it was irreversible.

My dear friend George Emerson pushed me to go to MD Anderson in Houston. He kept telling me they have equipment and techniques that no one else has, and that their clinical trials yield more results than others. My nephew Jason also encouraged me to get a second opinion, especially before undergoing irreversible surgery. He told me that he really encourages his patients to get a second opinion, because either it will confirm his diagnosis, or he will learn something new that only makes him better. I called MD Anderson (MDA) and began the process.

Sometimes the smallest step in the right direction ends up being the biggest step of your life.

Tiptoe if you must, but take the step. And what a step, what a process it was!

If there is any question that could ever be asked of a person about their medical history, MDA asked it in their pre-visit paperwork. I have never seen an organization that was so thorough. They also requested all scans, procedures etc., as well as all clinical notes from every doctor and hospital I had been to in the preceding five years.

Clara and I flew to Houston the next to last weekend in September. My cousin Jeff Williams, who I hadn't seen in over forty years, picked us up at the airport and took us out to dinner. Clara ordered the restaurants signature dish—gluten free fried chicken. She said it was the best she ever had. We had several meals with Jeff during the time we were there, and that reminded me so much that no matter what situation you are in, there is always, ALWAYS something to be grateful for!

We booked a stay at a very unique and eclectic hotel, only a few miles from MDA. We felt like we had stepped into a '60's avant-garde movie set. On Monday morning we took a shuttle to the hospital, and a new chapter opened in my journey. After taking care of the myriad of paperwork, we were brought back to meet the person who would be in charge of my care at MDA, Dr. Tina Cascone. She was born and raised in Italy, and in addition to a distinct accent, she also spoke so fast it was next to impossible to write down everything she said. The first thirty minutes she met us, she did not look at a single note or sheet of paper. I was amazed and commented on it. She said, "You can tell I spent my weekend getting to know you." I told her that was obvious, and that I had spent my weekend getting to know her. When she looked at me quizzically, I told her where she was born, where she went to college, where she went to medical school, where she had interned, done residency and fellowships. She said, "I have never had any patient know so much about me, especially before I even met them!" I told her that my life was literally in her hands, and I wanted to know whose hands I was putting my life in! We formed a bond then and there. I make sure to send her a CD with all images after any scan, along with all notes and interpretations. She often calls me out of the blue, saying she was thinking about me. When Clara and I went to California I bought her an angel Christmas tree ornament because she literally was my angel.

In February 2020 I was able to check off the next to last item on my original bucket list as I led 47 people on a pilgrimage to the Holy Land. In Bethlehem we bought her a hand carved olive wood pocket cross that I mailed her along with the disk from my most recent scan. She called me the night of March 30, 2020 to tell me how much it meant to her, how the smell reminded her of growing up in Italy, and that her husband said we must really know her! It is so wonderful to meet a person who is doing exactly what they were created to do, and Dr. Cascone is certainly that.

Dr. Cascone scheduled me for a brain MRI, along with a thoracic oncology consult on Wednesday, a full PET scan, and MDA was sending off tissue from my first lung surgery (which they received from VCU) for a full molecular profile. They also asked me if they could bank tissue and blood samples for future researchers to study. I was the recipient of many others who had done the same thing before me, so I readily agreed, firmly believing the day you plant the seed is not the day you eat the fruit. People from all over the country, indeed from all over the world, come to MD Anderson, usually for a second opinion like mine. MDA knows how to get everything scheduled in just a few days. They are truly one of a kind! When we met with Dr. Cascone on Tuesday before all the tests, she called me the "superstar" of her clinic. By that she meant that I had already beaten two deadly cancers and she thought what I had was going to be "cured with a pill." I wasn't sure I heard her correctly, but Clara said that was what she heard too.

Clara and I wandered around the streets of Houston with our carry-ons on our backs and wheeling our luggage, looking very much homeless. We were in a very well to do neighborhood with fabulous homes and well-kept yards and gardens. We jokingly said it would be so nice if someone would take pity on us and invite us in for cheese and crackers. We happened upon a little café/coffee shop named Coco, and knew it was for us. For years Clara and I would end each text message to each other with "xoxo" which autocorrect would change to "coco." Eventually we stopped using xoxo altogether and just used coco. When we saw it was a bakery/coffee shop/café we knew where we were was where needed to be. And that one little thing, finding Coco, made all the difference in the world. It felt like the universe was sending me/us a message and that we were indeed where we needed to be. The drop in our anxiety was palpable.

I said from the first day of diagnosis, and repeated it many times in the subsequent days. If you want to beat cancer, you have to BELIEVE, down to the molecular level of your being that you *are* going to beat it, no matter what! You can't just think you might, or that maybe you'll have a chance. NO! You have to convince yourself, down to the very molecules that make up who you are, that if one in a million beat this, it will be you. Convince every cell in your body, and then believe it with all the power of your mind. Our minds are the most power-ful tools in our arsenal, yet many people fail to fully harness their potential, simply because they don't try, or don't try hard enough, or give up.

I had a breath prayer I would do every night before going to sleep. I would lie in bed, slowly breathe in as deep as I could while thinking the words, "Breathe in healing," After holding my breath (the healing) in for as long as I could, I would then slowly exhale and think the words, "Breathe out cancer." I stayed focused solely on that and pushed all other thoughts out of my head and kept doing it until I fell asleep.

Have you ever been unable to recall someone's name, but an hour or two later you suddenly blurt it out, even though you're no longer actively seeking that information? That is your mind, working in the background, on a task you left it to do. Many inventions have come about because the person working on it got stuck and went to bed. Sometime during the night or the next morning they awoke with a start and had either solved the impasse or had gone in a different direction that allowed them to later. The answers you seek never come when the mind is busy, they come when the mind is still. If I cut my finger, I can't just heal it. But actually, yes, I can! My brain doesn't know how to heal the cut, but my mind does. Your body's ability to heal is greater than anyone has permitted you to believe. I've always felt the strongest argument for God is our body's ability to heal themselves. If my body could heal a cut or mend a bone, then surely it could rid me of this cancer if I gave it the right tools, meaning the right medicines, the right doctors, and an absolute positive belief that I would prevail.

"In deep and lasting ways, when we heal ourselves we heal the world."~Mark Nepo

On October 1, 2018, less than a week after my first visit to MD Anderson Dr. Cascone's colleague, Dr. James Allison, won the Nobel Prize in Medicine. His work revolutionized cancer treatment by determining how to disengage the "brakes" that prevent the immune system from attacking cancer. His discoveries led to a new class of drugs called checkpoint inhibitors that now form the fourth pillar of cancer treatments, along with surgery, radiation and chemotherapy. Dr. Allison studied a protein that previously had been identified as a restraint on the immune system. There was a possibility that I would be a candidate for Dr. Allison's study, based on one entry Dr. Cascone had read in the first pathology report about the removal of my right upper lobe. We would conclusively know when the molecular profile report came back.

As humans we can deal with the known much better than we deal with the unknown. Even if the known turns out to be something really bad, like terminal cancer. Knowing for sure what we are facing produces less stress and anxiety than not knowing.

Clara, the kids and I were thrust back into that realm of

crushing anxiety because of not knowing. I have always dealt with stress by being super functional. The more things are out of my control, the more I deal with the things I can control. Catherine Pulsifer once wrote, "One of the best lessons you can learn in life is to master how to remain calm."

We were scheduled to travel to MD Anderson a second time on October 31, 2018 for a week of testing, discernment and decision making about the next stage and course of treatment. The Staff Parish Relations Committee at Chester United Methodist Church, where Clara was the new senior pastor, unanimously passed a resolution giving her the freedom to go to all appointments with me, whether in Richmond or in Houston, and that her full salary and benefits would be paid and the time away would not be considered vacation. This was one of the greatest gifts anyone had ever or could ever give us. The Administrative Board also passed it unanimously. This is the church being the church. When Clara was with me at appointments, she felt guilty about not giving her all to Chester. When she was at work, she felt guilty about not being with me. It was the ultimate Catch-22. Now the church had taken both the pressure and the anxiety and the guilt away. It truly was a gift of unselfish love, one we will remember and cherish forever.

We went back to Houston October 30th. The joy this time was we were picked up at the airport by a young man who now lived and worked in Houston, but who had been a member of our church and youth group at Saint Luke's. We took Lucas out to dinner and then he graciously took us to the grocery store. We did a better job of selecting where to stay this time by renting an Airbnb with a full kitchen.

The next day I had a long day of tests and consultations. A little after 4:00 PM we got to the interventional radiology consult. The main reason we went to MDA this second time was because we were told they had the best technicians in the world to do biopsies. Even the thoracic surgeon we met with on the prior visit said as much. He said he also worked at the Mayo Clinic, and that he didn't have anyone there who was able to correctly biopsy areas as small as a certain technician at MDA could do. My team at Massey desperately wanted the lymph node under my left clavicle biopsied. I learned later that the lymph node under the collarbone on the opposite side of the primary tumor is one of the first things doctors look for to determine if the cancer has spread.

During the consultation, the nurse talked about the next day's procedure on my right lung. About fifteen minutes into it I asked her why she wasn't also telling me about the left lymph node. She looked through all her paperwork, consulted my chart and even left the room to make a phone call. When she came back, she informed us that the thoracic surgeons determined it was too small to biopsy. I was both crestfallen and a little angry. The entire reason we paid for plane tickets to Houston, a place to stay for a week, was because my team at Massey did not feel they had anyone who could successfully biopsy that node, but MDA assured us they could. I told the nurse about this, and then we *really* got to see the incredible efficiency of MDA. Clara and I left the consultation and began walking the half mile or so to the Thoracic unit. I had them on my cell phone and had a hard time hearing them and I know they had a hard time hearing me because of my labored breathing from walking as fast as I could. Thankfully the entire walk was inside as a torrential rain was happening outside.

It was not too long removed from Hurricane Harvey which had devastated the Houston area, and as we walked, we could see the concrete spillways rising rapidly through the windows. We got there before the unit closed at five o'clock, even though I had to stop several times on the way and rest my hands on my knees to try and catch my breath. In the waiting room I got three calls in succession on my cell phone, and just like that, an attempt was going to be made to do an ultrasound guided biopsy of the left lymph node in the morning at the same time as my already scheduled one for my right lung, and MDA had also made sure insurance would cover it. If you've ever tried to make an appointment for something like this, waited on hold until someone finally answered and then were given a date weeks or months in advance you can appreciate the excellence, speed, and professionalism of MDA. Some people there literally moved heaven and earth in order for me to get both biopsies!

Dr. Cascone had already arranged for a complete schedule of care to treat what we thought was Stage III neuroendocrine lung cancer. She was visibly shaken when she saw our suitcases in the exam room and I let her know we were heading back home to Chesterfield where I was going to have Massey Cancer Center coordinate my care with her. She reluctantly understood, as most patients who come to MDA for diagnosis return home for treatment.

On Tuesday of that week, she had presented my case to the tumor board at MDA, comprised of the chairs of every medical specialty that takes care of patients there. Included on that board was Dr. James Allison.

After presenting the result of my biopsies, the tumor board was surprised at the results. Neuroendocrine carcinoma, indicating a recurrence of the lung cancer from the previous year, but it also showed features of adenocarcinoma, and according to the tumor board, they had never before seen this particular arrangement of different cancers in the same tumor. I wrote on Caring Bridge that I wasn't sure if I liked or didn't like being "unique" to the tumor board at MD Anderson.

The decision was made to send these tissue samples off for molecular testing. Dr. Cascone called my thoracic oncologist at Massey, Dr. Erin Alesi, and also me. She frantically wanted to make sure I hadn't started any chemotherapy at all. If I had, it would disqualify me for immunotherapy. Thankfully I had not, and we anxiously awaited the results of the genetic testing. If the testing came back that I was ALK+ or that the ALK gene had rearranged on the surface of the tumor, then I would qualify for a medicine developed from Dr. Allison's groundbreaking discoveries. If not, it meant I would need to go to Houston for three days every two weeks for 4-6 cycles and then be placed in a double-blind study. Once again, it was time to hurry up and wait.

On November 27, 2018, Dr. Cascone called with the news. The little sample of tissue they obtained from the biopsy on November 1 came back showing an abnormal rearrangement of the ALK gene (ALK+). We all have 2 pairs of 23 chromosomes for a total of 46. These chromosomes contain all of our DNA which encodes the genetic information that is a blueprint of all proteins and other similar molecules that perform all of our cellular functions. Sometimes part of a chromosome known as a gene (which encodes a specific protein) can develop a mutation, and this can produce a protein with altered function since its blueprint was altered by the mutation. In other situations, parts of the chromosome can become deleted, duplicated, or even flip/invert within itself, all of which can distort genes or even lead to new abnormal genes and any of these changes can lead to new or abnormal proteins. Most of the time, these types of changes don't do anything damaging, or if they do are able to be recognized as bad by the cell and then killed to prevent a problem to the body. However, sometimes these changes can make a cell become capable of growing uncontrollably and resistant to dying.

In ALK+ lung cancer, part of chromosome #2 inverts within itself and fuses together 2 particular genes that are not normally next to each other—these genes are called EML4 and ALK. ALK on its own plays a role in normal cell growth and proliferation and is known as a "tyrosine kinase protein" which we all need in normal cell activities. However, when ALK is fused together with EML4, the new fusion protein that it produces results in uncontrolled activation and constant growth, leaving the cell unable to stop. This is what leads it to become a cancer.

Alectinib or Alecensa is a type of drug known as a tyrosine kinase inhibitor, TKI for short—it is a drug that specifically binds to and blocks ALK's ability to activate the cell and therefore stops its growth. Nowadays, there are many different types of TKIs that have been developed to target different cancers that have similar types of abnormal proteins like ALK. They have completely transformed the way we are now able to treat patients with these diseases.

In the write up from my original lung surgery (remember at the time of surgery we didn't know what the spot was), Dr. Cascone had read one short sentence indicating the tissue sample may be ALK+. Talk about thorough! And even though the neuroendocrine and adenocarcinoma together in the same tumor had only been reported *twice* in all the medical literature, and was never ALK+, Dr. Cascone convinced the tumor board to send off these biopsies for molecular testing. She shakes her head and disagrees when I call her my angel, but she truly is! More than likely, I would not be here writing this book if it had not been for Dr. Cascone. Sometimes God will use your deepest pain to launch your greatest calling. I believe that is what has happened to me. Just because I carry it all so well doesn't mean it's not heavy. A good friend said to me,

**"One day you will tell your story of how you've
overcome what you're going through now, and it will
be part of someone else's survival guide."**

And it's not just me. I would say to every person who reads this book—Someone, somewhere, is depending on you to do what God has called you to do. Katherine MacKenett said it best,

"Now, every time I witness a strong person, I want to know. What dark did you conquer in your story? Mountains do not rise without earthquakes."

It was the best possible news. I wasn't going to have to go back and forth to Houston, I could be treated at home. The tumor board at both Massey *and* MDA were extremely invested in watching to see how my progression played out as the combination of cancers together with the re-arrangement of the ALK gene had not been seen in the medical literature before. Any time a situation like this occurs, we have a chance to "move the needle" closer to a cure. Even though what I was going through I wouldn't wish on anyone else, I was given yet another opportunity to "pay it forward" and help those who would come after me. It wasn't the first time in my life I had this happen.

When I was a graduate student at Duke University, I took a position as a Resident Advisor to help finance that expensive education. RA's act as house parents to undergraduates. In exchange for the University provided room, RA's maintain order, offer help when they can and are the link between the on-campus students at large and the administration. Duke University liked to use older graduate students in these roles as much as possible, feeling they would be more mature and perhaps even a little intimidating to the undergraduates. The Divinity School at Duke offers magnificent "field placement" (sort of like clinicals for nurses, or residencies for doctors) where one could earn enough money over a 10- or 13-week summer placement to cover all first semester costs except housing. Being an RA really helped to lower the high cost of seminary education at Duke. Being older than most grad students, and being in the Divinity School, I was asked to take on the role of Area Coordinator. In that position I oversaw the entire East Campus of Duke, with all the dorms, RA's and students. My field placement had ended a few days before the doors were supposed to open for RA training so I was basically homeless for a few days. I called the student housing office and made the argument that since they were entrusting me to oversee all these dorms, RA's and students, could I be trusted to move in a few days early? That way I would be settled and could better help the new crop of RA's move in themselves and get somewhat adjusted before all the students arrived.

They agreed and I began moving into my room on the second floor. Housekeeping was getting the dorm ready for the year, and they were sanding and refinishing the hard wood floor in the commons room on the first floor. I had two big glass lamps carried football like in my right arm, and a framed picture of Buffalo NY in my left. If you approach Buffalo in the air from Lake Erie, the harbor looks just like an American Buffalo, hence its name. I slipped on the fine layer of sawdust that covered the marble steps and fell hard! On my way down my mind was racing a thousand miles an hour which slowed down time. I twisted my body as I was falling so that I wouldn't break the picture of Buffalo, and in so doing the entire weight on my body crashed onto my right arm carrying the lamps. They broke and with my entire weight behind them acted like cleavers. I had cut off my entire right hand, except for the bone. Blood was spurting everywhere and I immediately screamed for help. My father had committed suicide June 16, 1985 by slitting his wrist and I identified his body. I did not want to die the same way as my dad. As Providence would have it, just as I tripped and fell two people came in to the building. Edna Andrews was the Russian language professor and had a faculty in residence space on the ground floor of Alspaugh dorm where I would be living. With her walked her boyfriend from high school, Mike. Mike was a medic in the Marines, took one look at me and knew what to do. He sat me down, wrapped a towel around my arm and helped me hold it higher than my heart. I was losing quite a bit of blood, but he kept me laughing, which kept me awake until the ambulance came.

Once in the hospital, they were able to stop the bleeding and assess the damage. All the nerves, blood vessels and tendons were completely sliced through. I had indeed cut off my hand except for the bone. Not sure how to proceed, the emergency room doctors called the chief orthopedic surgeon, Dr. James Nunley, and asked him what to do. Nunley was such a sought-after surgeon that his calendar was booked months, even years in advance for certain surgeries. After listening to the report of what happened, he told them he had a cancellation for 7:30 the next morning and would take me. Dr. Nunley along with another doctor in Australia had just pioneered a new surgery for injuries such as mine, and was anxious to see if it would work.

A nurse that spoke to Clara was so calm and reassuring that Clara didn't speed during the five-hour ride to get to Duke from her placement. We were planning our wedding for the following summer and she was busy with that. Clara's eyes got as big as saucers when the doctor tested my feeling by poking me with a card that had two points and would ask "how many points" did I feel each time he went up and down my arm and hand. I never answered, as I never felt anything. That was when she knew it was serious.

The only thing I remember about the surgery was the anesthesiologist putting a mask over my face and asking me to count backwards from ten. When I got to four, Dr. Nunley started taking off the gauze and wraps from the night before. I reached up with my left hand, lifted the mask and said, "I'm not out yet!" I was in so much pain I just needed him to wait a few more seconds before he began.

The surgery to put me back together took quite a few hours, as there was a *lot* to do. When I came to in the recovery room, I remember feeling like my arm was wound so taut that I wondered if I was even getting blood flow. A little later when the initial pain meds wore off, I felt much different sensations.

I worked as hard as I possibly could during physical therapy for close to a year. After 2100 hours or more of physical therapy I was able to regain all the movement in my right hand and fingers, although not all of the feeling. The surgeon who put my hand back together told me it was the first time someone regained independent flexor movement (moving each finger individually down to be able to touch the tip of the finger to the palm of the hand) after a zone five injury. Remember, when I was a child, my mother would say to me, "Your problem is you don't know when to quit." Well, I didn't quit when I was working to regain the use of my hand, and I wasn't going to quit fighting now.

In 1941, Franklin Roosevelt declared December 7th as a "day that will live in infamy." It was for me and my family, as December 7, 2018 is when I began the Alectinib therapy.

That Christmas Eve was the first time in thirty-two years that I was not presiding over Christmas eve services. It was difficult to sit in the balcony of Chester UMC as a congregant rather than upfront as the worship leader. However, sitting with three of my children was also something I had never done during Christmas Eve services, so the trade-off was worth it!

As I sat there waiting for the birth of the Christ child again, I thought these thoughts, and my prayer that evening for all my children was this:

May all that has been reduced to noise in you, become music again.

On the way home from Christmas Eve service, I heard Rick Warren founder of Saddle Back Church say these words,

"Other people are going to find healing in your wounds. Your greatest life messages and your most effective ministry will come out of your deepest hurts."

I was no longer lamenting not leading worship, I was rejoicing being with my children and the feeling I had found my next calling—writing this book. Don't forget—the day may come when you are the lighthouse in someone else's storm.

9

The Past is in Your head.
The Future is in Your Hands

*When you're going through hard times and wonder where
God is, remember the Teacher is always silent during the test.*

*If you want to know where to find your contribution
to the world, look at your wounds.
When you learn to heal them, teach others.*

2019 started off with the news that squamous skin cell cancer
had been found (again) on my right temple. I had known that
something was there for months, and was finally able to get in
to see the dermatologist. It was going to have to be removed
by MOHs surgery. This is a process where they keep taking
away layers of skin around the site until they are comfortable
they got what is considered safe margins. When they do, the
surgery is considered curative.

Because of how toxic Alecensa is, I have to have a weekly
blood draw. The numbers from my kidney function were too
high, almost to the point of having to stop or alter the medicine.
I wrote that on my Caring bridge site, and a former member
of my church wrote that her sister was on the same medication
and was having the same issue. To help your body process the
medication, it is recommended to drink an abnormal amount
of water throughout the day, which I had been doing. Lori said

her sisters doctor discovered that too much water was actually harmful, and she recommended drinking a sports drink for half the liquid. Products like Gatorade and similar drinks have far too many sugars in them, but Body Armor does not. I did that and at the next blood draw my total bilirubin (which measures liver function) was in the normal range, my conjugated bilirubin was only 0.1 above normal, the best numbers I had posted since starting on the Alecensa. My doctor also had a blood panel run and my total cholesterol was the lowest it's ever been, my "good" cholesterol was the highest it's been, and my triglycerides were at an all-time low. Diet, exercise, and a sound suggestion from a similar journeyer, and the ship was righted.

Ryan and his Dutch girlfriend Marije (whom we affectionately call our "daughter-in-love") came in from Holland on March 8, 2019 and it was the first time I was able to be with all four of my children at the same time since my 60th birthday celebration in January of the previous year. When your children are younger you take for granted everyone sitting at the dinner table every night. As they grow up and move out you realize just how sacred these family times around the table are.

The following week was going to be the most important week I had since undergoing the bone marrow transplant. I was scheduled for my first full CT scan since I had started on Alecensa. I had been warned at MD Anderson that many patients have a much worse first CT scan after their baseline, due to the cancer trying to fight back against the ALK inhibitor. The day after the scan I was scheduled to have my first chemo infusion since starting the drug, and no one really knew what to expect as there was not much data in the medical literature about how Alecensa and Rituximab interact. I joked to some friends that if I were a landfill, I'd probably be banned in 35 states for being so toxic. I wrote on Caring Bridge, "I can sleep tonight knowing there are people who are much smarter than me looking at every single variable and every single interaction and balancing this living chemistry experiment that I have become." I wouldn't wish what I've gone through on anyone and my hope is that my experience will move the needle in the direction of a cure.

Usually, the combination of drugs they give me "on board" before infusing the Rituxinab keeps me wired for days, but at the same time just listless with no energy. I decided I needed to do all I could do to change that. I was going to have the honor of presiding at my lifelong best friend Chris Cauley and his fiancée Karen's wedding the next week down in Key West, so I went out and bought myself new clothes for that. I went to the grocery store to buy the fixings for making an epic dinner for Clara. I walked 5 ½ miles and then blew all the leaves off our 1.2-acre property. Later that night after Clara had gone to bed, I lost myself for over three hours on the piano.

If you've ever known someone with lung cancer, they will tell you it is painful. Sometimes more than others. For whatever reason, the time I'm describing above was one of the most painful times. I was as diligent as I could be to show as little as possible of this to Clara, but I also refused to take any pain medicine. I reminded myself that the only organism that can feel pain is a live one, and the pain was just a reminder that I was in fact, still alive.

On March 15th we got the results from the first post-Alecensa CT:

NO new growths!

Some tumors had disappeared!

The largest tumor had shrunk from 1.6 CM to under 0.5 MM!

I just could not imagine any better results. I told Clara on the way home I feel like someone who has been told their entire life that they could not have a child, but then miraculously discovers they are pregnant.

The side effects of the medication are brutal. I don't talk about these except with Clara and my doctors. I don't put them on Caring Bridge or tell my kids about them. It really takes a toll on your liver. I have a blood test every two weeks, and my bilirubin numbers are usually too high. They will get to the point where we think we might have to do something different, and then I'll pop off a good test or two so we stay status quo. The medication also gives me fatigue that can be severe at times. Unless you've had chronic fatigue you don't know what it's like. Sleeping 8–10 hours or even getting a long nap doesn't help. You wake up as tired as when you fell asleep. There have been times when I haven't been able to make it all the way up the steps without stopping to rest. I do try to keep these to myself so my family isn't overly worried.

Dehydration is a constant companion, but weirdly, at the same time the medication causes me to retain a lot of fluid, particularly in my abdomen and extremities. Every exam the doctor checks these and asks about it. My hands had swollen to the point that my wedding band was so tight it was starting to cut off the circulation. I really didn't want to take it off because I had never taken it off, even for a minute, from the moment Clara put it on my finger on our wedding day.

Our children have taught us that anyone can learn to do anything just by watching YouTube videos. My wedding band had never been taken off, my finger had gotten thicker over the years, as had my knuckle, and now my hand and fingers were swelling as well. In addition to the ring being stuck, I had developed a condition my dermatologist called "ring rot" where the skin and muscle were actually dying. The ring had to come off.

Clara and I decided we could do it ourselves by watching a few YouTube videos. If Brandon could teach himself how to replace a ball joint on his truck by watching a video, surely we could be taught some easy method of removal we hadn't thought of yet. Several videos showed rubbing Vaseline deep into the finger, and then carefully winding dental floss around the finger tighter and tighter until the ring could just easily slide off. I'll spare the gruesome details but suffice it to say it didn't work for me like it did for the folks who made the video. The tightly wrapped floss caused me to lose almost all circulation and I was afraid I might lose my finger. Far from helping, when we finally got the floss off, the finger swelled even more. We didn't learn our lesson the first time but tried a couple more times, all with the same result. You know what is said about doing the same thing over and over and expecting different results?!

Finally, I did it the old-fashioned way. I just pulled on it and smoothed out the skin whenever it bunched up and after forty-five very painful minutes it finally came off. It had been on 10,844 days. Clara offered to buy me a new one but I refused. I found a jeweler in town who could resize it and I took it to them. Three weeks later the ring rot had healed and I put my ring back on. Now I have to see if I can wear it 10,845 days and break my record.

One time a few years back Taylor talked with me about going sky-diving someday. We talked about it a few times but never actually got around to doing it. It's always good to have hopes and dreams and plans for the future. They can keep you going in dark valleys. But it's also important to act on them, so realized hopes and dreams and plans become part of the makeup of your spiritual DNA.

Taylor's birthday was coming up on April 1. If you know Taylor, you know that is the perfect day for him to have as his birthday. I told Taylor I would like to take him and Hannah skydiving and any of our other children that wanted to go.

Ryan and Marije were in Holland so they were out. Brandon our risk taker extraordinaire surprised me by saying he wasn't interested, and deathly afraid of heights—Clara said no way. That left Laura. At first, she said no, but reconsidered it for a few days and said if I called the skydiving center and they had room, that was the universe telling her to jump. If there was no room it meant the universe was saying don't go. I called and there was room and so early one Saturday Taylor and Hannah, Laura and I head to the Virginia Skydiving center in Wakefield, VA.

It was a ton of fun! We each had our own jump buddy. This person is certified in tandem jumping and does all the work. All you have to do is scream and have fun. I also paid extra so we each could have our own videographer who jumped with us and recorded everything. This person flew around like Batman, and got video and pics from above, below and in front. It was amazing. When the plane gets to the right altitude, you start scooching towards the door, with your jump buddy securely strapped to your backside. Then you are almost completely dangling, with only the instructor/jumper still in the plane and when you nod you are ready, they push off in free fall. They intentionally barrel roll you a few times to see how strong your stomach is, before the instructor pulls a cord for a tiny parachute to release, which does nothing to slow your free fall, it just aligns you in the upright position.

The pressure on my ears drums was astounding, as was the noise of the air rushing by my ears. It is quite a weird feeling to be free falling to Earth! Then the instructor pulled the cord to release the main chute, and all fell silent. Eerily silent. And beautiful! You get a view of earth you've never seen, and hope-fully a new perspective as well. After all, isn't that the purpose of a new view in life, to allow you to see a different perspective? The instructor started making long slow turns so we could be in the air longer and pointed out things on the ground I might not recognize. Down in the landing field I did recognize Taylor and Hannah as they had gone on a flight before Laura and I. Then I had to do the second and last job of the jump. The first job was to get my ankles together and both my legs as far under and behind me as I could, making sure they were between the instructor's legs at all times as we were dropping. As we approached landing, I was supposed to bring them in front of me, keep them together, and lift them as high as I could, like a gymnast. The instructor explained numerous times that if my feet hit the ground before his, we would tumble wildly all over the place and get wrapped up in the chute. If I kept my legs straight and together and off the ground until his hit first, we would have a picture-perfect landing. I did, and we did, and it was beyond awesome! To see so much exuberant joy pouring from Taylor, Hannah and Laura made it all worthwhile. On the way home we talked about how we wanted to do it again. When I showed our videos and pictures to Clara, she got jealous enough that she said she thought she might like to try it too someday. We will see! It reminded me of the lyrics of a popular country song by Tim McGraw that often played on the radio:

"He said
I went skydiving
I went Rocky Mountain climbing
I went 2.7 seconds on a bull named Fu Manchu
And I loved deeper
And I spoke sweeter
And I gave forgiveness I'd been denying
And He said
Someday I hope you get the chance
To live like you were dying"

In May I had my every other month Rituxin infusion. Because

of all the medication that is put "on board" before I receive the actual Rituxin, I usually spend two days without sleep and have zero energy. But for some reason this time around it was the opposite. Clara had been wanting a raised bed vegetable garden ever since we moved in. I surprised her for her birthday by building her one out of lumber left over from when the previous owners had the fence installed. The day after infusion five yards of topsoil was delivered and I transferred it all, wheelbarrow load by wheelbarrow load into the garden. Then I power-washed the entire area around my pool and did the same with the hot tub. Then I vacuumed the pool. In all that day I put over 21,000 steps in, which is a little over ten miles. I surprised even myself, and it truly gave me hope for the future of what life could be like when I had energy.

Then came the three-year anniversary of being told I had lymphoma. I reflected on it a lot that day. I wouldn't wish what I'd be through on anyone, and yet I still wouldn't change anything about what happened. You can't control what happens to you, you can only control your actions and reactions, and there is where your power lies. I was a better person, a better husband, a better father, a better Christian and a better pastor. The lymphoma found the lung cancer and because it did, I'll be eternally grateful I got the lymphoma. Clara describes it as a higher state of being. We were able to travel to California where I had the honor of presiding over my best friend Bruce's wedding to his beautiful soul-mate Kellie. Clara and I rented a BMW convertible and drove both the Avenue of the Giants (redwoods) as well as US1, the Pacific Coast highway. Along the way I took over one hundred pictures of flowers. After being given less than a year and a half to live, I had stretched it to three and got to experience things I didn't think I ever would again. This is why you never, ever give up—Ever!

Father's Day 2019 came. And once again, it was on June 16th. My father took his own life on Father's Day, June 16, 1985. Every Father's Day has been bittersweet for me since I've been a father, because of that. But these feelings are particularly poignant when it again falls on June 16th. There is such a big part of me that just wants to celebrate with my four beautiful children and what wonderful people they are and another part of me that goes to the darkness and relives June 16, 1985, like a closed loop of self-inflicted pain.

I fought so hard the last six years just to live another day that it is beyond foreign to me to think about taking my own life. Yet as I get older, I think I understand my father better—his demons and his isolation. I used to hate my father for what he had done to himself, to my mother, to me and the rest of my family. I forgave him years ago when Clara made me understand that if I didn't, my children would probably never learn to forgive me, and the cycle would continue. As I once again stood on the precipice between life and death, I wondered yet again about his thoughts in his last moments of life. I remember saying, "I'm sorry, Dad, that the pain you felt inside was so incredibly deep that you saw no other option than to die. You live on in me, and in my children, who never got to meet you."

Be the person who breaks the cycle.
If you were judged, choose understanding.
If you were rejected, choose acceptance.
If you were shamed, choose compassion.
Be the person you needed when you were hurting,
not the person who hurt you.
Vow to be better than what broke you—to heal
instead of becoming bitter so you can act from your
heart, not your pain.
~Lori Deschene

The CT scan in July came back with mixed results. The good news was all the existing tumors and nodules remained stabilized. The bad news was a new nodule with "spiculated margins" showed up in my lower left lobe. It was small and we caught it early, but the spiculated margins were of concern as this indicated a cancer of some sort. It was too small to biopsy, and as always, talking on the phone with Dr. Cascone of MD Anderson helped lower both mine and Clara's anxiety. I remember lying in bed wide awake one night when Clara was asleep and saying out loud, "OK God, I got it. I learned the lesson/s. I promise you I won't forget them. Can we stop now?"

After consultation with Massey Cancer Center and MD Anderson, the decision was to take a conservative approach and wait and see, we scheduled a follow-up CT scan in September, a month early.

In the late spring/early summer I again began going into Afib regularly. About three or four times a week and often my heart rate would be 120-140 for hours. I remarked to numerous people that it felt like I had run a marathon except my legs weren't tired. My cardiologist had me wear a heart monitor for a number of weeks, and with this information was able to convince the insurance company that I needed to do a heart ablation. During the procedure, the surgeon goes into the heart through a large vein in the leg, and freezes the tissue where the faulty signals originate.

Everything coalesced in September. I had the follow-up CT scan on the fourth, my bi-monthly Rituxin infusion on the fifth, a consult with my primary doctor on the ninth, heart Ablation surgery on the eleventh, and a follow-up with my pulmonologist on the thirteenth, and a colonoscopy on the twentieth! I jokingly told a friend that September was, "Keep every medical specialty in business month." For me it was!

Normally the radiology report can take up to a week to

come back, so I was surprised the afternoon of the fourth that my oncologist was calling. I was very apprehensive answering the phone, she had never called the same day as the CT before. But she called to tell me that she was amazed. Not only had the report come back sooner than anyone expected, but the new nodule that appeared in my left lung was gone, with only a residual "ghost trace." She said the wording in the report was surprisingly positive because they tend to err on the side of caution, but it was a glowing report, as much as a CT scan can be. We were even able to cancel our trip to MD Anderson, and the travel agency got my tickets refunded in full.

Everything seemed to be falling my way, and for that, I was indeed thankful!

I am not what has happened to me. I am what I choose to become.
~C.G. Jung

Never Give Up, Never Ever Give Up.

Today is a great day to be alive.

Go do something today for someone who is fighting for their tomorrow.

Life is short, enjoy it while you can.

DO WHATEVER IS NEXT

Epilogue

Listen to silence, it has much to say. ~Rumi

The quieter you become, the more you can hear

I was able to check off the last two items on my bucket list—to go to the Holy land again, and to be free from my medi-port. It is February, 2022 now, and I am thrilled to say I led a group of 47 pilgrims in February 2020. We returned to the States just as the Covid pandemic was beginning. The last item was also one of symbolic significance. I wanted the medi-port removed from my chest. That would be the very real and tangible evidence that I had in fact, been the one in a million to beat MCL, and just before I went to the Holy Land, that was done. It has taken me that long to write and edit this book. At some point this book has to end, and I don't want that to coincide with my life, so here it is. If I live long enough, I'll write a sequel. If I don't, YOU write the sequel!

I have metastatic cancer, meaning it will never be cured. Last week (2/18/2022) we switched from Alecensa (Alictinib) to Lolatinib (Lorbrena) because the ALK gene had mutated a second time and outsmarted the first drug. The Alecensa gave me over three years, so here's hoping I get the same on the Lorbrena before I have to switch again.

At this point I don't know how my story will end. But I do know one thing it will never say is: **He Gave Up**

Acknowledgments

Clara and I set up a Caring Bridge site, mainly so that we wouldn't have to answer the question "How are you doing?" 600 times every Sunday. It's humbling to me that at the time of this writing there have been over 75,000 visits to that site, and so the first acknowledgment simply has to be to all of you who come read the updates after every alert. I have read every single comment ever left, most of them multiple times. I look at the list of names of those who visited and pray for each of you by name, because YOU have become my primary source of strength, and your encouragement to write this book is why it is now written.

One of those visitors to my site was Pat Murphy. Pat had been a member of Saint Luke's before moving to Norfolk, VA where she plies her trade as a graphic designer. Pat offered to help bring this book to fruition, and she has. Than you Pat! This wouldn't have crossed the goal line without you.

Bishop Charlene Kammerer, Rev. Bass Mitchell, Dr. Michael Marcum, and Dr. Omid Safi all read this while it was still a manuscript and all provided wonderful feedback. Any and all mistakes herein are mine alone, but this is a stronger book because of the above four.

About the Author

Doug Gestwick grew up in Western New York where he became a life long Buffalo Bills fan and long time member of the Bills mafia, —Go Bills! He received his undergraduate degree from SUNY Geneseo, where he was to meet his life long mentor and friend Leonard Sweet. After college he sold computers for seven years before realizing that wasn't for him, and applied to, and was accepted into Duke University Divinity School. In addition to earning a Masters of Divinity and Master of Theology Degree, Doug caught the eye of an incoming first year, Clara Price, and they married while she was in her last year of the M.Div program, and he was completing his ThM. Becoming United Methodist pastors meant entering into an itinerant system, and they settled into the Virginia Conference. Between them they served 10 churches over a 33 year ministry. It was at the next to last Church, in Bridgewater, Virginia, where they learned to work together in the same church and for many years they were the only clergy couple serving together as Senior Pastor and Associate Pastor at the same church. When it was time to leave Bridgewater, they asked the Bishop to please send them to a church where they could stay at least eleven years so that their four children could all have the same high school diploma and not have to move during those turbulent teen years. They ended up staying twelve years living with, and ministering among, the wonderful people of Saint Luke's in Yorktown, Virginia. It was there Doug discovered he had mantle cell lymphoma, and this incredible journey began.

Doug and Clara now live and play out of their beautiful oasis home in Chesterfield, VA along with his other faithful companion Argo, a 15 year-old black lab that often thinks she is still a puppy.